Auditory System - Function and Disorders

Edited by Sadaf Naz

Published in London, United Kingdom

Auditory System - Function and Disorders
http://dx.doi.org/10.5772/intechopen.98024
Edited by Sadaf Naz

Contributors
Alex Hoetink, Huib Versnel, Nathan van der Stoep, Gijsbert van Zanten, Wiepke Koopmans, Juan Bautista Calero del Castillo, Alberto Guillen Martinez, Francisco Garcia Purriños, Ahmad Aidil Arafat Dzulkarnain, Nur Hafizah Sulaiman, Fatin Amira Shahrudin, Shahrul Na'im Sidek, Hazlina Md. Yusof, Madihah Khalid, Milaine Dominici Sanfins, Caroline Donadon, Piotr Henryk Skarzynski, Maria Francisca Colella-Santos, Wlodzimierz ("Vlad") Wojcik, Alexandros-Apostolos A. Boulogeorgos, Stylianos E. Trevlakis, George K. Karagiannidis, Sadaf Naz, Ayesha Imtiaz, Bint-e- Zainab, Alishbah Sheikh, Kanwal Shabbir, Zunaira Munir, Hina Khan, Hifza Idrees, Memoona Ramzan

First published in London, United Kingdom, 2022 by IntechOpen
IntechOpen is the global imprint of INTECHOPEN LIMITED, registered in England and Wales, registration number: 11086078, 5 Princes Gate Court, London, SW7 2QJ, United Kingdom

British Library Cataloguing-in-Publication Data
A catalogue record for this book is available from the British Library

Additional hard and PDF copies can be obtained from orders@intechopen.com

Auditory System - Function and Disorders
Edited by Sadaf Naz
p. cm.
Print ISBN 978-1-80355-189-0
Online ISBN 978-1-80355-190-6
eBook (PDF) ISBN 978-1-80355-191-3

Meet the editor

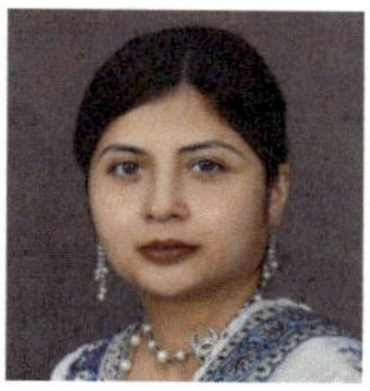

Professor Sadaf Naz is a geneticist who received her Ph.D. in Molecular Biology from the University of Punjab, Lahore for her studies on recessively inherited deafness in Pakistan. She conducted post-doctoral research at the National Institute on Deafness and Other Communication Disorders (NIDCD), National Institutes of Health (NIH), USA on the genetics of hearing loss in humans and animal models. In 2005, she was appointed as a faculty member at the School of Biological Sciences, University of Punjab. Her research interests encompass the genetics of moderate-to-severe hearing loss, movement and neurodevelopmental disorders, skeletal dysplasias, as well as psychiatric disorders using conventional genetic methods or massively parallel sequencing.

Contents

Preface

The auditory system is a complex organ that perceives sound, converts it into electrical signals, and conveys these signals to the brain for interpretation. The various cells in this system are arranged to form an extremely intricate architectural structure. The functions of these cells in the auditory system are equally diverse. Their roles are mediated by a vast plethora of different protein components. Given the high complexity of the structure and function of the auditory system, it is not surprising that multiple things can and do go wrong. Malfunctions of the auditory system can affect any of its parts. The outer ear can be deformed or missing. Middle ear development can be impaired. These defects may result in conductive hearing loss. However, by far the most common defect is sensorineural hearing loss, which is due to inner ear dysfunction. This book discusses the different structures and functions of the auditory system in both normal and impaired hearing.

The first section of the book presents the basic structure of the auditory system. Chapter 1, "Structure and Physiology of Human Ear Involved in Hearing" presents the gross organization of the ear. It describes various cell types and the acellular membrane in detail. Chapter 2, "Electrophysiology and Auditory Training," discusses the recording of electrical changes collected through electrodes placed on the scalp as a tool to help in monitoring auditory intervention programs.

The second section includes three chapters related to auditory brainstem responses. Chapter 3, "Short Latency Evoked Potentials of the Human Auditory System," discusses auditory brain stem responses. Chapter 4, "Precocious Auditory Evoked Potential Recording with Free-Field Stimulus," describes a case series study of children assessed by auditory brain stem responses as well as auditory steady-state responses. Chapter 5, "Auditory Brainstem Response with Cognitive Interference in Normal and Autism Spectrum Disorder Children - Understanding the Auditory Sensory Gating Mechanism," presents findings concerning auditory brain stem responses with cognitive interference in healthy children and auditory sensory gating capacity in those with autism spectrum disorders.

The third section deals with the genetics of hearing loss. Chapter 6, "A Short Overview on Hearing Loss and Related Auditory Defects," describes different inherited deafness forms as well as the very common age-related hearing loss. Chapter 7, "Nonreceptor Protein Kinases and Phosphatases Necessary for Auditory Function," discusses those protein kinases and phosphatases variants that are known to cause hearing loss in humans or mice.

The final section defines cochlear prosthetic devices and optical wireless cochlear implants. Chapter 8, "Issues in Creation of Bio-Compatible Cochlear Signal: Towards a New Generation of Cochlear Prosthetic Devices," highlights problems and suggests solutions for the treatment of hearing loss. Finally, Chapter 9, "Hearing Restoration through Optical Wireless Cochlear Implants," presents two new implant architectures for improving the efficiency and reliability of hearing-restoration devices.

I would like to thank Commissioning Editor Ms. Lucija Tomicic-Dromgool and Author Service Manager Ms. Sara Debeuc at IntechOpen for their help throughout the publication process.

Sadaf Naz,
School of Biological Sciences,
University of the Punjab,
Lahore, Pakistan

Section 1

Structure and Physiology of the Auditory System

Chapter 1

Structure and Physiology of Human Ear Involved in Hearing

Alishbah Sheikh, Bint-e-Zainab, Kanwal Shabbir and Ayesha Imtiaz

Abstract

Hearing is the fundamental sense based on the normal functioning of the hearing organ "the ear," which plays a vital role in social interaction and the ability of learning. The human ear is divided into three parts: the outer, middle, and inner ear. Defects in outer and middle ear can cause conductive hearing loss, while the defective inner ear may lead to sensorineural hearing loss. So, it is important to study the structure and physiology of the human ear. When a sound of particular frequency enters the outer ear, it passes through the auditory canal and strikes the tympanic membrane. It vibrates and passes these vibrations to three ossicles present in the middle ear. The ossicles amplify the vibrations of sound and send them to the cochlea in the inner ear. Cochlea contains organ of Corti, which converts these vibrations into electrical signals by its hair cells. The neural signals in turn are interpreted by the brain, which one can hear and understand. The aim of this chapter is to review the basic structure and physiology of different parts of the human ear that are involved in the hearing process.

Keywords: hearing, human ear, organ of Corti, auditory system

1. Introduction

Sound is a mechanical energy wave which can travel through in air or any other physical medium (gas, liquid and solid). These longitudinal waves consist of alternating compressions and refractions. When sound waves travel through a medium, the particles of that medium vibrate parallel to the direction of sound wave that explains the longitudinal wave nature of sound. A human speaker or any other sound source produces the specific vibration patterns that are converted into appropriate auditory signals by the ear [1].

Hearing is the fundamental sense that allows one to perceive the sound. It also helps the person to communicate and detect different environmental signals. Human ear converts the physical vibration (sound) into a nerve impulse which is further processed by central auditory pathway of the brain. This mechanism of the sound interpretation is complex [2]. This chapter will mainly discuss the structure of different parts of the ear and their physiological interplay in hearing.

IntechOpen

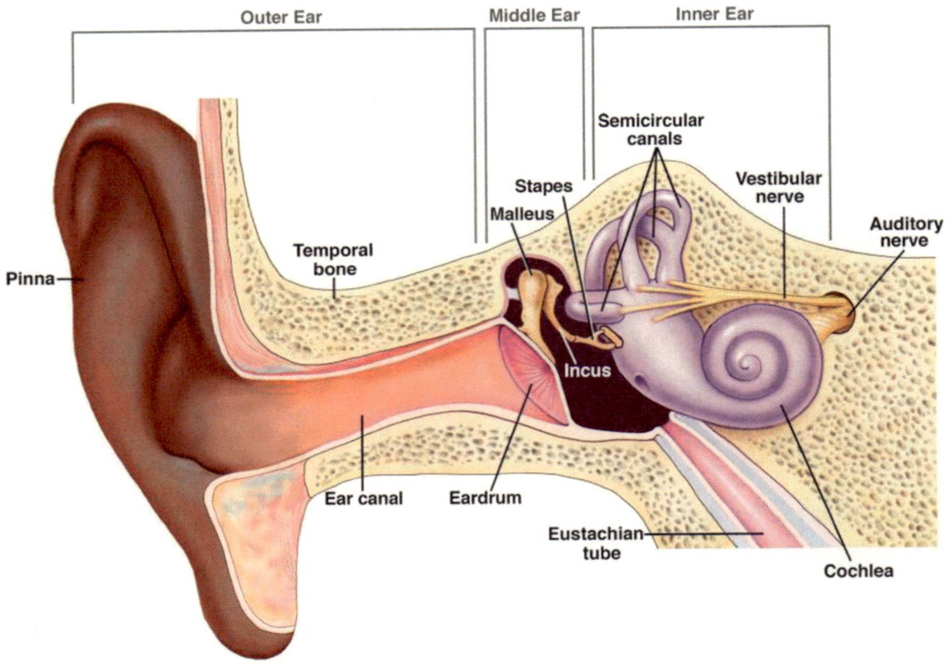

Figure 1.
Structure of the mammalian ear. The ear is partitioned into three parts: Outer, middle, and inner which are shown here. The outer ear contains the pinna, ear/auditory canal, and the tympanic membrane which separates it from the middle ear cavity. The middle ear is linked to the back of the nose by the Eustachian tube and contains ossicles known as malleus, stapes, and incus. The inner ear is divided into vestibular labyrinth and cochlea. The vestibular labyrinth further contains semicircular canals and the vestibule (source NIDCD, with permission).

The hearing organ "the ear" is a paired organ, located one on each side of the head. Each ear contains the cochlea, a snail-shaped coiled moiety, as the sense organ. A human ear has hearing range of 20–20,000 Hz through the air conduction while this range is greater for much higher frequencies in case of bone conduction. The former part of the ear deals with conducting the sound to the sense organ cochlea and then the cochlea is responsible for the transduction of vibrations, which is performed by delicate hair cells. The ear is structurally and functionally partitioned into three parts that are required for normal hearing: the outer inner, middle ear, and the inner ear—the latter is further divided into the vestibular labyrinth and cochlea (**Figure 1**). These are discussed in detail below.

2. Structure and physiology of outer ear

The outer ear comprises the pinna and the auditory canal both of which transmit the focused sound signal on the tympanic membrane which separates the outer ear and middle ear. For functional hearing, proper development of the outer ear is essential. As outer ear defects are involved in a number of syndromic and non-syndromic conditions of conductive deafness, it is very crucial to understand the structure of the outer ear [3].

2.1 Pinna

The pinna protruding from the side of the skull is comprised of cartilage and is completely covered with skin. It is responsible for collecting the sound vibrations and funneling them to the auditory canal. The pinna is helpful in localizing the sound as it catches the sounds, which are more efficiently coming from the front than those coming from behind because of its angle. But this effect is applicable only in the case of high frequencies because of the wavelength of audible sound vibrations and also the relative size of the head. The head itself has a role in localizing the sound as it casts a shadow of sound in the case of middle frequencies, and in lower frequencies, the phases of sound arrival between the ears are responsible for localizing the sound.

2.2 Auditory Canal

The auditory canal is about 4 cm in length and the outer part with hairy skin and the inner thinner part (**Figure 1**). The outer hairy part has sebaceous and sweat glands [4, 5], both of which together with keratin form ear wax. The ear wax and the hair growth in the outer part of the canal serve as a disinfectant and provide a protective barrier for the ear. Moving inward, the skin of the auditory canal is thin and it is firmly attached to the deeper ear canal bone, which is a hard cavity that absorbs faint sound and then directs it to the tympanic membrane at its base.

2.3 Tympanic membrane

The tympanic membrane has an outer layer of skin that is continuous with the auditory canal and an inner layer called the endoderm [6]. The outer ectodermal layer is made of stratified and squamous epithelium, which displays lateral unique migration of cells from the center to the edges of the tympanic membrane where these epidermal cells can then exfoliate [7]. This process is referred to as the self-cleaning property of the outer ear. The inner layer of the tympanic membrane comprises of a simple squamous epithelium [8].

The tympanic membrane is divided into two main regions based on its morphology (**Figure 2**); firstly, the tense structure appropriate for the vibration known as the ventral pars tensa, and second the more elastic one the dorsal pars flaccida.

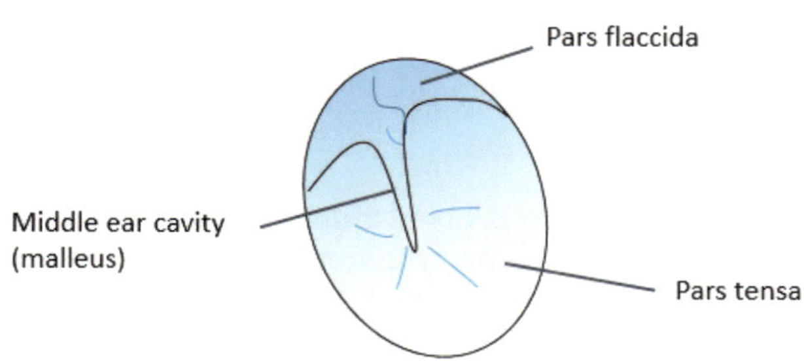

Figure 2.
The structural morphology of the tympanic membrane. Schematic of tympanic membrane, which is partitioned into two parts based on morphology: One the pars flaccida and second the pars tensa.

The pars flaccida also called as Shrapnell's membrane is in the upper part of the tympanic membrane above the malleolar fold and is a relatively more fragile region than the other larger part of the tympanic membrane, the pars tensa [8, 9]. Both of these regions are tri-layered structures containing an inner layer of neural crest cells, which are in the arrangement of loose connective tissue, and this middle layer is sandwiched between two epithelium layers. The inner layer of pars tensa is the lamina propia consisting of further two collagen-rich connective tissue layers [10]; the outer radiative layer and an inner circular layer. While in pars flaccida there is no regular arrangement of extracellular matrix in the inner layer. So, both these regions of the tympanic membrane, the pars tensa and pars flaccid, are different from each other at a cellular and gross level. These structural and functional differences explain why retraction pocket (a condition in which the tympanic membrane is pulled more deeply into the middle ear cavity and may cause pain) more commonly occurs in pars flaccida [11].

The whole tympanic membrane structure has a thickness of about 0.1 millimeters and in the middle ear cavity, it covers an opening (round) of about 1 cm in diameter. Although the tympanic membrane is generally referred to as the eardrum, technically the middle ear cavity is the eardrum with the tympanic membrane acting as the drum skin [12].

3. Structure and physiology of middle ear

The middle ear, an air-filled cavity is associated with the back of the nose by a long and thin tube known as the Eustachian tube (**Figure 1**). In the middle ear, the outer wall is the tympanic membrane while the cochlea is the inner wall. The middle ear floor is a thin bony plate that covers the beginning of the jugular bulb, a great vein that drains the blood from the head. At the upper limit of the middle ear, it forms the bone beneath middle lobe of the brain. At the middle ear front end, there is the opening of the Eustachian tube, and at its posterior end lies a passageway to mastoid cells, which are a group of air cells present within temporal bone [12]. The middle ear, lined with the respiratory membrane, is basically an extension of respiratory air spaces of the sinuses and the nose. This respiratory membrane, thick at the Eustachian tube and thin when passing through mastoid, can produce mucus [13]. The Eustachian tube is a bony structure as it leaves the middle ear but, in the nasopharynx, comprises of cartilage and muscle. The tube is opened by active contraction of muscles which also allows to equalize the air pressure in both the middle ear and nose.

3.1 Auditory ossicles

The middle ear contains three small bones: malleus, incus, and stapes (also commonly known as hammer, anvil, and the stirrup, respectively, (**Figure 1**)). These ossicles conduct the sound from the ear drum to the inner ear. The malleus is club-shaped with its handle buried in the tympanic membrane, running along its center to upward, and its head lying in the middle ear cavity above the tympanic membrane where it is suspended through a ligament from a bone that forms brain covering. Here, the head of a club articulates with a cone-shaped incus. The base of cone articulates with the malleus head, above the tympanic membrane. The incus, present between two other ossicles, has a thin projection protruding out from it called as its long process. It freely hangs in the middle ear and is connected to stapes at its tip which has a bend of right-angle. The third ossicle stapes is an arch-shaped bone comprising a footplate and an arch. The footplate is articulated by the joint of the stapedio-vestibular as it covers the oval window which is an opening into the vestibular system of inner ear or cochlea [14].

4. Function of outer and middle ear

To understand the role of the outer and middle ear in hearing physiology, it is important to first study the conducting mechanism of sound. The audible sound range is about 10 octaves from somewhere between 16 and 32 Hz to somewhere between ~16,000 and 20,000 Hz. The sensitivity of sound is above 128 Hz to ~4000 Hz and this range of maximum audibility and sensitivity decreases with age. As mentioned earlier, the head itself forms a natural barrier between the two ears. This plays a role in sound localization based both on the intensity and the difference in time of arrival of sound. Moving to the pinna, its crinkle shape catches and funnels the high frequency sounds to the auditory canal, which acts as a resonating tube since it amplifies the sounds falling between 3000 and 4000 Hz to increase sensitivity of the ear at these respective frequencies. The ear responds to very low-intensity sounds owing to its sensitivity. The equal pressure of air on both sides of the tympanic membrane also enables this sensitivity. The Eustachian tube provides this equalized pressure by opening for short intervals with every 3rd or 4th swallow. If it remained open all the time, one could even hear the sound of his or her own breath. If the Eustachian tube is closed for too long; it can absorb oxygen and carbon dioxide from the air in the middle ear. As the middle ear comprises lining of a respiratory membrane that can absorb gases, this process produces negative pressure. This may cause pain as is the case during descent of an airplane if the Eustachian tube is not unblocked. The middle ear cavity is quite small, containing mastoid air cells which act as air reservoirs to provide the cushion effects to pressure change. If the negative pressure remains for too long then the fluid is secreted by the middle ear cavity, which can cause conductive hearing loss [12, 15].

The outer and middle ears amplify the sound signal since the pinna has a relatively large surface area and funnels the sound to smaller tympanic membrane which has in turn large surface area as compared to the stapes footplate. This results in hydraulic amplification [16] i.e., a smaller movement over a large area is being converted into larger movement to a smaller area. The ossicular chain acting as a lever system amplifies the sound. Overall, both the outer and middle ears amplify the sound by about 30 dB on its passage from outside to the inner ear.

5. Inner ear

The human inner ear is present between the middle ear and acoustic meatus and is labeled as a labyrinth of ear that can be a bony or membranous labyrinth that each is further divided into three portions. Bony labyrinth comprises of semicircular canals, the vestibule, and the cochlea whereas the membranous labyrinth comprises of the semicircular duct, two sac-like structures of the vestibule; namely the saccule and the utricle and the cochlear duct (**Figure 1**). The space between the membranous and bony labyrinth is filled with watery fluid named perilymph that is obtained from the lymphatic system, and it is similar but not identical to the aqueous humor of eyes and cerebrospinal fluid. It is poor in potassium and rich in sodium ions [17, 18]. Membranous labyrinth also has enclosed fluid named endolymph, which has a high potassium concentration, and its composition is different from that of perilymph. Endolymph is produced by vestibular dark cells that have a resemblance with stria vascularis, which is part of the cochlea [18]. Endolymph within the membranous labyrinth of inner ear interacts with hair cells and causes depolarization of hair cells by providing high potassium gradient, resulting in afferent nerve transmission [19]. These structures form two systems of inner ear, a vestibular system involved in maintaining equilibrium and the cochlear system only part of the ear that participates in hearing. The vestibular system is proprioceptive (feedback loop between sensory organs and nervous system, external stimuli is not involved in it), whereas the cochlear system is exteroceptive (sensation in cochlea is caused by external stimuli e.g., sound).

5.1 Vestibular system

Many hearing loss disorders are accompanied by vestibular defects, which necessitate some description when considering the auditory system. The vestibular system is a sensory system of inner ear that is important for postural equilibrium maintenance and helps develop coordination between the position of the head and eye movements. It comprises of five organs; three semicircular canals that are present at right angles to each other and control angular (Head) rotation and two otolith organs that play a vital role in linear acceleration (straight line movement) [20]. Semicircular canals based on their position are designated as superior, posterior, and horizontal. Each canal opens into the vestibule through its expanded end known as Ampulla. Sensory neuroepithelium in ampulla is known as crista ampullaris consisting of ridge of tissues. From cristae arises a gelatinous protein-polysaccharide structure, cupula that divides the ampulla into equal parts and is important to keep hair cells in place [21]. Rotational acceleration causes endolymph to displace cupula which results in bending of hair cells in direction opposite to acceleration [22]. It is the middle part of bony labyrinth that is connected posteriorly with the semicircular canal and anteriorly with the cochlea and separated through the oval window from the middle ear.

Two membranous structures of the vestibule are the utricle and saccule are designated as otolith organs [22]. A single patch of sensory neuroepithelium in the vestibular system is called macula, which is present on the inner surface of a membranous sac. It lies in the utricle in the horizontal plane and originates from the anterior wall of the tubular sac. Whereas in saccule it is in the vertical plane and covers the bone of the vestibular inner wall. Gelatinous otolithic membrane (macula) of utricle and saccule contains thousands of otoconia (calcium carbonate crystals) embedded in a protein matrix [23]. In mammals, these otoconia are arranged to form various layers that help the hair cells to respond to endolymph drag. The sensory cells in vestibular region are hair-like cilia that project out from the apical end that are flexible motile kinocilia and stiff non-motile stereocilia. The stereocilia are arranged according to curvilinear line called striola [24], the area of thickening of saccule and thinning of utricle [25]. If the endolymph pressure is toward the kinocilium; it causes opening of cation channel and potassium influx resulting in depolarization of hair cells. This depolarization of hair cells results in release of glutamate to afferent nerve receptors and neurotransmission. Various signals from the vestibular nucleus are sent to the cortex, thalamus, and cerebellum that in return send efferent signals to the ocular and postural muscles [26].

5.2 Cochlea

Cochlea is a coiled hollow bony structure that is lined by epithelial tissue. Despite being a bone, it is requisite for hearing and transduction as part of the auditory system. It is named after the Greek word 'kokhliās', meaning snail, due to its coiled shape (**Figure 3A**). This spiral shape of the cochlea helps it to differentiate between different frequencies because the different but specific region of the cochlear spiral detects different frequencies. Cochlea consists of three canals lined by epithelial cells that are filled with fluids. It also has the organ of Corti, which is a sensory organ that converts sound energy into neural signals that are conducted through the nerve fibers to the brain [29–31].

5.2.1 Canals of cochlea

Cochlea consists of three canal systems (**Figure 3C**); the scala vestibuli, the scala media and the scala tympani which envelop the modiolus. These three scala wind around the bony axis in a spiral stairway.

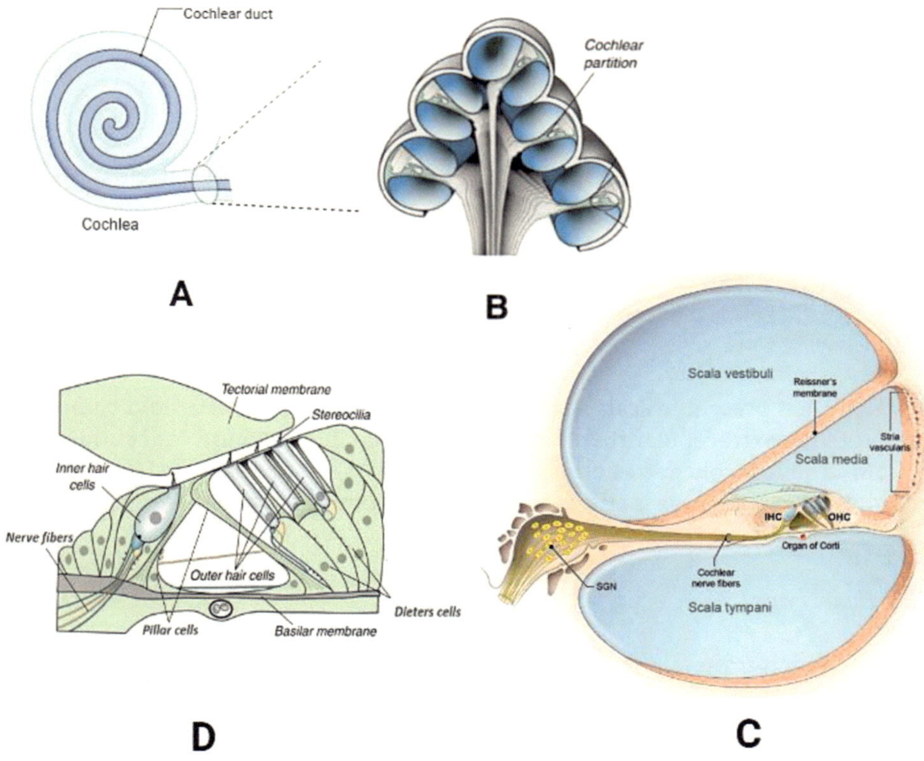

Figure 3.
Cochlear anatomy. A. Cochlea Structure. B. Cross-section of cochlear duct showing fluid-filled cavities around the modiolus. C. Three main canals: Scala vestibuli, scala tympani, and scala media along with Reissner's membrane, stria vascularis and the organ of Corti in middle. D. Magnified view of the organ of Corti, containing outer and inner hair cells, stereocilia and supporting cells with tectorial and basilar membranes (taken from [27, 28] with permission).

5.2.1.1 Scala vestibuli

Scala vestibuli is the exterior lymph-filled canal and it is connected to the vestibules of the inner ear. The oval window is present at the base of the scala vestibuli. It is the part of cochlea that receives vibrations from the middle ear (stapes). Scala vestibuli and scala tympani sense the change in pressure that is caused by the different frequencies of sound.

5.2.1.2 Scala tympani

Scala tympani is the inferior canal and it connects to the tympanic membrane forming the two-and-half coiled structure of cochlea. Its superior end is connected to the scala vestibuli, while its inferior end separates the cochlea from the round window. The point at cochlear apex where scala vestibuli and scala tympani meets is known as the helicotrema.

5.2.1.3 Scala media

Scala media is present between the scala vestibuli and the scala tympani and has the organ of Corti and the basilar membrane. A basilar membrane is present between the scala media and the scala tympani, thus separating them. Scala media also contains the spiral ganglions that are extended neurons from the hair cells. The stria vascularis of scala media is involved in the regulation of K^+ into scala media, thus maintaining the potential of endo-cochlea [32].

5.2.2 Fluids of cochlea

The chambers of the cochlea are filled with three types of fluids: perilymph, endolymph, and intrastrial fluid. These fluids maintain the endo-cochlear potential which is important for sensory transduction. The intrastrial fluid only fills the cavities present in stria vascularis.

5.2.2.1 Perilymph

Perilymph is present in scala vestibuli and scala tympani, and its fluid composition is similar to the extracellular fluid of the body. It has a high sodium concentration (140 mM) and low concentration of calcium (1.2 mM) and potassium (5 mM). The perilymph present in scala media is continuation from CSF while that in scala media is from plasma of blood.

5.2.2.2 Endolymph

Endolymph is present only in the scala media and has a unique ionic composition i.e., high K^+ concentration (150 mM), which is not found anywhere in the body. This high concentration of K^+ helps to maintain the endo-cochlear potential. Hence, endolymph is a noteworthy characteristic of the cochlea. It has considerably low concentration of sodium (1 mM) and calcium (0.002 mM) [32–34].

5.2.3 Reissner's membrane

Reissner's membrane is present between the scala vestibuli and scala media and is involved in the regulation of ions. The membrane along with the basilar membrane creates a cavity in the cochlear duct that is filled with endolymph. It is an avascular membrane that is made up of two types of cells. The part of Reissner's membrane cells that lines the scala vestibuli are fibroblasts, while the cells that line scala media are epithelial cells. This cavity also contains the sensory organ i.e., the organ of Corti. Two types of ion channels are present on Reissner's membrane: potassium ion channel and non-selective cation channel. These channels maintain the pressure between endolymph and perilymph [35, 36].

5.2.4 Organ of Corti

The organ of Corti is the organ for audition and is present on the basilar membrane. It consists of outer and inner hair cells (mechanosensory cells) and supporting cells (**Figure 3D**). The organ of Corti hair cells also has stereocilia that attach it to the tectorial membrane (soft ribbon-like structure on the top of organ of Corti). Alterations in basilar and tectorial membrane help in the movement of stereocilia that stimulates the hair cell receptors [37–39].

5.2.4.1 Tectorial membrane

The tectorial membrane covers the mechanosensory and supporting cells of organ of Corti. It has a viscous structure consisting of collagen and non-collagen proteins (glycoproteins and proteoglycans). The membrane helps in storing the calcium ions for the sensory organs of the inner ear. The stereocilia present in the organ of Corti are embedded in the tectorial membrane [40].

5.2.4.2 Mechanosensory cells

The hair cells are erect and contain micro-projections at their apical ends, known as stereocilia, that are filled with F-actin. The arrangement, size, and toughness of the hair cells in the cochlea are responsible for responding to different ranges (low to high) of sound frequencies. The cochlea shows a fundamental effect of tonotopy. Tonotopy refers to the orderly coding of sound based on high to low frequencies by hair cells and their afferents (spiral ganglion neurons). The hair cells residing at the apex of cochlea reciprocate to lower frequencies while the ones at the base, near to oval window reciprocate to a higher range of frequencies, thus creating a tonotopic gradient all over the cochlea. The hair cells convert the sound energy into neural signals.

5.2.4.2.1 Outer hair cells

Outer hair cells are oblong cells containing myosin and actin protein, which help these cells contract in rhythmic movement in response to sound stimuli from the middle ear. There are about 12,000 outer hair cells that are arranged in three rows. At the top of these cells are stereocilia that are embedded in the tectorial membrane. These cells are present on the basilar membrane area where the largest frequencies would be received [41]. These cells play a role in mechanoelectrical stimulation as well as in the feedback mechanism for low-frequency sounds for its amplification. They can amplify the faint sound by the inversion transduction through the positive feedback mechanism i.e., conversion of electrical signals to mechanical (sound) signals. The outer membrane of outer hair cells has a unique motor protein known as prestin, which is involved in the generation of movements that couple back to the wave produced in a fluid membrane. In this way, weak sounds are amplified by the 'active amplifier' mechanism [42, 43].

5.2.4.2.2 Inner hair cells

The primary organ for the audition is the bundle of inner hair cells. These cells have pear-shaped morphology, and their stereocilia make weak connections with the tectorial membrane. There are about 3500 inner hair cells arranged in just a single row that is surrounded by supporting cells. These hair cells transmit the electrical signal to the auditory cortex of the brain through the nerve fibers. About 95% of auditory nerve projection to the brain is through inner hair cells. The outer hair cells help inner cells in the generation of synaptic nerve conduction to cochlear nerve fibers [37].

5.2.4.2.3 Supporting cells

Supporting cells are rigid sensory epithelial cells, organized in a mosaic manner that during the head movement and stimulation of sound maintain the integrity of the sensory hair cells. These cells play a vital role in maintaining the microenvironment for the proper functioning of hair cells. There are different types of these cells that are arranged in a row on the basilar membrane. They are Hensen's cells, Deiters' cells (phalangeal cells), pillar cells, Claudius cells, Boettcher cells, and border cells. These are arranged from the outer edge to the inner edge of an organ of Corti. These cells maintain the structure of the organ of Corti as well as the composition of the endolymph in the scala media. Supporting cells have negative resting potential so these cells tend to transport Na^+ out and K^+ into the scala media through the channels present in these cells [44, 45].

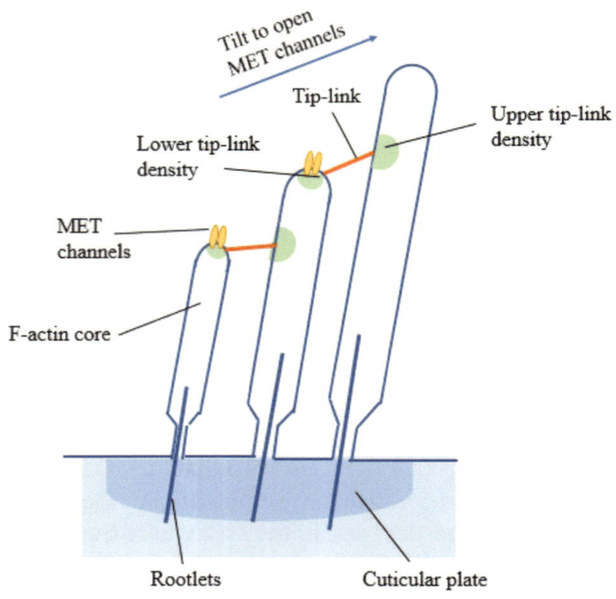

Figure 4.
Structure of stereocilia on hair cells. The stereocilia are made of F-actin protein and these stereocilia are linked to each other through the tip links. When the largest stereocilium moves due to the pressure at the tectorial membrane, the shorter ones move as well and mechanotransduction channels (MET channels) open and influx of ions takes place.

5.2.5 Mechanotransduction in cochlea

A small number of transduction channels present in the stereocilia are open at the resting state. The stereocilia consist of shafts of F-actin protein, which has upper and lower tip link densities that help in linking the long and short stereocilia through tip links (**Figure 4**) [46]. These stereocilia are arranged in ascending order of their height. When the largest stereocilium embedded in the tectorial membrane is displaced, the ones with shorter lengths also move. These movements of stereocilia open the mechanotransduction channels present at the tips of the stereocilia, leading to an influx of K^+. As a result, the voltage-gated calcium ion channel opens and uptake of Ca^{2+} into the cells takes place. This depolarization of cells excites the cochlear nerves and in turn, results in the release of glutamate from the hair cells into the auditory nerves. The sound wave signal is then conveyed to the brain. Both the apical and basal regions of the cochlea are separated by membranes and their extracellular ionic environments are tightly regulated. These regulations of ions are important for converting the sound signals into electric impulses that are sent to the brain [47].

6. Conclusion

The human ear, one of the most developed sensing organs, has structurally and functionally divided into three parts. Firstly, the outer part, containing pinna and auditory canal, passes the sound vibrations to the tympanic membrane which separates the outer and middle ear. The middle ear containing the three ossicles (malleus, incus, and stapes) receives these vibrations and amplifies them. Traveling through middle ear, the vibrations are passed to inner ear which contains the spiral-shaped cochlea as the sense organ. In cochlea, the hair cells present in the organ of Corti contain stereocilia whose rhythmic movements open the mechanotransduction channels, which send the nerve signal to the brain. In this way, these vibrations are converted into understandable sound.

Acknowledgements

The authors thank Inna A. Belyantseva and NIDCD, NIH, USA, for permission to use figures in this chapter.

Author details

Alishbah Sheikh†, Bint-e-Zainab†, Kanwal Shabbir† and Ayesha Imtiaz*
University of the Punjab, School of Biological Sciences, Quaid-e-Azam Campus, Lahore, Pakistan

*Address all correspondence to: ayesha.sbs@pu.edu.pk

† Authors have equal contribution to this chapter.

References

[1] Rahman A, Hoque ME. Harvesting energy from sound and vibration. Retrieved from Researchgate Net. 2013;**90**:166-171

[2] Moore BC. An introduction to the psychology of hearing. Brill. 6th ed. 2012. pp. 34-55

[3] Anthwal N, Thompson H. The development of the mammalian outer and middle ear. Journal of Anatomy. 2016;**228**(2):217-232

[4] Perry ET, Shelley WB. The histology of the human ear canal with special reference to the ceruminous gland. The Journal of Investigative Dermatology. 1955;**25**(6):439-451

[5] Niemann C, Horsley V. Development and homeostasis of the sebaceous gland. Seminars in Cell and Developmental Biology. 2012;**23**(8):928-936. DOI: 10.1016/j.semcdb.2012.08.010

[6] Carlson B. Chapter 13. Sense Organs. Carlson, Human Embryology and Developmental Biology. 5th ed. Philadelphia, PA: WB Saunders; 2014. pp. 269-293

[7] Kuijpers W, Van der Beek J, Jap P, Tonnaer E. The structure of the middle ear epithelium of the rat and the effect of Eustachian tube obstruction. The Histochemical Journal. 1984;**16**(8):807-818

[8] Lim DJ. Tympanic membrane: Electron microscopic observation part I: Pars tensa. Acta Oto-Laryngologica. 1968;**66**(1-6):181-198

[9] Lim DJ. Tympanic membrane. II. Pars flaccida. Acta Otolaryngology. 1968;**66**(6):515-532

[10] Probst R, Grevers G, Iro H. Basic Otorhinolaryngology: A Step-by-Step Learning Guide. Vol. vii. New York: Georg Thieme Verlag; c2006

[11] Maw AR, Hall AJ, Pothier DD, Gregory SP, Steer CD. The prevalence of tympanic membrane and related middle ear pathology in children: A large longitudinal cohort study followed from birth to age ten. Otology & Neurotology. 2011;**32**(8):1256-1261

[12] Alberti PW. The anatomy and physiology of the ear and hearing. Occupational Exposure to Noise: Evaluation, Prevention, and Control. 2001;**1**:53-62

[13] Nuutinen J, Kärjä J, Karjalainen P. Measurement of mucociliary function of the eustachian tube. Archives of Otolaryngology. 1983;**109**(10):669-672

[14] Thompson H, Ohazama A, Sharpe PT, Tucker AS. The origin of the stapes and relationship to the otic capsule and oval window. Developmental Dynamics. 2012;**241**(9):1396-1404

[15] Luers JC, Hüttenbrink KB. Surgical anatomy and pathology of the middle ear. Journal of Anatomy. 2016;**228**(2):338-353

[16] Killion MC, Dallos P. Impedance matching by the combined effects of the outer and middle ear. The Journal of the Acoustical Society of America. 1979;**66**(2):599-602

[17] Sterkers O, Ferrary E, Amiel C. Production of inner ear fluids. Physiological Reviews. 1988;**68**(4):1083-1128

[18] Echteler SM, Fay RR, Popper AN. Structure of the mammalian cochlea. In: Comparative Hearing: Mammals. New York: Springer; 1994. pp. 134-171

[19] Ciuman R. Stria vascularis and vestibular dark cells: Characterisation of main structures responsible for inner-ear homeostasis, and their pathophysiological relations. The Journal of Laryngology & Otology. 2009;**123**(2):151-162

[20] Ekdale EG. Form and function of the mammalian inner ear. Journal of Anatomy. 2016;**228**(2):324-337

[21] Mescher A. Chapter 23. The eye and ear: Special sense organs. Junqueira's Basic Histology: Text & Atlas. 14th ed. 2016. pp. 499-522

[22] Barrett K, Barman S, Boitano S, Brooks H. Chapter 10. Hearing & Equilibrium. Ganong's Review of Medical Physiology. 24th ed. New York: McGraw-Hill; 2012

[23] Zhao X, Yang H, Yamoah EN, Lundberg YW. Gene targeting reveals the role of Oc90 as the essential organizer of the otoconial organic matrix. Developmental Biology. 2007;**304**(2):508-524

[24] Tascioglu AB. Brief review of vestibular system anatomy and its higher order projections. Neuroanatomy. 2005;**4**(4):24-27

[25] Oghalai JS, Brownell WE. Chapter 44. Anatomy & physiology of the ear. In: Lalwani AK, editor. CURRENT Diagnosis & Treatment in Otolaryngology—Head & Neck Surgery, 3e. New York, NY: The McGraw-Hill Companies; 2012

[26] Kingma H, Van de Berg R. Anatomy, physiology, and physics of the peripheral vestibular system. Handbook of Clinical Neurology. 2016;**137**:1-16

[27] Tona R, Lopez IA, Fenollar-Ferrer C, Faridi R, Anselmi C, Khan AA, et al. Mouse models of human pathogenic variants of TBC1D24 associated with non-syndromic deafness DFNB86 and DFNA65 and syndromes involving deafness. Genes. 2020;**11**(10):1122

[28] Frolenkov GI, Belyantseva IA, Friedman TB, Griffith AJ. Genetic insights into the morphogenesis of inner ear hair cells. Nature Reviews Genetics. 2004;**5**(7):489-498

[29] Dallos P, Fay RR. The Cochlea. Vol. 8. Switzerland: Springer Science & Business Media; 2012. pp. 435-502

[30] Patuzzi R, Robertson D. Tuning in the mammalian cochlea. Physiological Reviews. 1988;**68**(4):1009-1082

[31] Slepecky NB. Structure of the mammalian cochlea. In: The Cochlea. New York, NY: Springer; 1996. pp. 44-129

[32] Dallos P. The active cochlea. Journal of Neuroscience. 1992;**12**(12):4575-4585

[33] Nin F, Yoshida T, Sawamura S, Ogata G, Ota T, Higuchi T, et al. HIBINO H: The unique electrical properties in an extracellular fluid of the mammalian cochlea; their functional roles, homeostatic processes, and pathological significance. Pflügers Archiv-European Journal of Physiology. 2016;**468**(10):1637-1649

[34] Ghanem TA, Breneman KD, Rabbitt RD, Brown HM. Ionic composition of endolymph and perilymph in the inner ear of the oyster toadfish, Opsanus tau. The Biological Bulletin. 2008;**214**(1):83-90

[35] Duvall AJ, Rhodes VT. Reissner's membrane: an ultrastructural study. Archives of Otolaryngology. 1967;**86**(2):143-151

[36] Raphael Y, Altschuler RA. Structure and innervation of the cochlea. Brain Research Bulletin. 2003;**60**(5-6):397-422

[37] White HJ, Helwany M, Peterson DC. Anatomy, head and neck, ear organ of corti. In: StatPearls [Internet]. Treasure Island, FL: StatPearls Publishing; 2021

[38] Lim DJ. Functional structure of the organ of Corti: A review. Hearing Research. 1986;**22**(1-3):117-146

[39] Kimura RS. The ultrastructure of the organ of Corti. International Review of Cytology. 1975;**42**:173-222

[40] Freeman DM, Masaki K, McAllister AR, Wei JL, Weiss TF. Static material properties of the tectorial membrane: A summary. Hearing Research. 2003;**180**(1):11-27

[41] Frolenkov GI, Atzori M, Kalinec F, Mammano F, Kachar B. The membrane-based mechanism of cell motility in cochlear outer hair cells. Molecular Biology of the Cell. 1998;**9**(8):1961-1968

[42] Ashmore JF. A fast motile response in Guinea-pig outer hair cells: The cellular basis of the cochlear amplifier. The Journal of Physiology. 1987;**388**:323-347

[43] Ashmore J. Cochlear outer hair cell motility. Physiological Reviews. 2008;**88**(1):173-210

[44] Glueckert R, Pfaller K, Kinnefors A, Rask-Andersen H, Schrott-Fischer A. Ultrastructure of the normal human organ of Corti. New anatomical findings in surgical specimens. Acta Oto-Laryngologica. 2005;**125**(5):534-539

[45] Bodian D. Electron microscopic atlas of the simian cochlea. Hearing Research. 1983;**9**(2):201-246

[46] Belyantseva IA, Labay V, Boger ET, Griffith AJ, Friedman TB. Stereocilia: The long and the short of it. Trends in Molecular Medicine. 2003;**9**(11):458-461

[47] Denk W, Holt JR, Shepherd GM, Corey DP. Calcium imaging of single stereocilia in hair cells: Localization of transduction channels at both ends of tip links. Neuron. 1995;**15**(6):1311-1321

Chapter 2

Electrophysiology and Auditory Training

Milaine Dominici Sanfins, Caroline Donadon,
Piotr Henryk Skarzynski and Maria Francisca Colella-Santos

Abstract

Electrophysiology is an objective evaluation method that allows investigating the responses of the central auditory nervous system arising from the capture of neuronal responses through surface electrodes. In addition to the possibility of investigating and diagnosing different pathologies, electrophysiology proves to be an effective and effective instrument in monitoring auditory intervention programs. Auditory rehabilitation programs is based on the premise of neuroplasticity that derives from a capacity for neuronal change due to intense sound stimulation, specific and directed to the patient's needs. Throughout this chapter, current studies that correlate electrophysiology with auditory training programs in different clinical populations will be presented, such as: hearing in typically developed individuals, hearing and school difficulties, hearing and CAPD, hearing and otitis media, hearing and hearing loss, and hearing and voice. Electrophysiological tests are important objective measures in predicting the gains to be expected from auditory training programs.

Keywords: auditory processing, electrophysiology, auditory training, auditory evoked potential, auditory rehabilitation

1. Introduction

Central auditory processing (CAP) refers to the processes involved in the analysis and interpretation of auditory stimuli. It encompasses the perceptual processing of auditory information by the central auditory nervous system and the neurobiological activity underlying it that gives rise to auditory evoked potentials. It is a well-defined and consolidated entity, both from a clinical and research point of view, as well as in terms of its disorders and associated diagnosis and rehabilitation. In this chapter, we describe aspects of CAPD, including its diagnosis through behavioral and electrophysiological testing. We will cover auditory rehabilitation procedures such as auditory training, and monitoring procedures which include the analysis of electrophysiological findings.

2. Central auditory processing disorder

Central auditory processing disorder (CAPD) is a deficit in "the perceptual processing of auditory information in the central nervous system (CNS) and the

IntechOpen

neurobiologic activity that underlies that processing" [1]. CAPD affects the perceptual and neural processes in the CNS which underlie sound localization and lateralization, auditory discrimination of speech and nonspeech signals, auditory performance when there is competing or degraded acoustic information, a variety of auditory temporal processing and patterning abilities, as well as others [2].

CAPD diagnosis can be performed at any age group, from childhood to adulthood. Alterations present in childhood may persist into adolescence and adulthood, may result from an acquired CNS event (traumatic brain injury, cerebrovascular accidents) and as part of the natural aging process. The estimated prevalence of CAPD may vary across age groups. In school age children the prevalence ranges from 2 to 5% [3] as a primary diagnosis. In cases where the CAPD co-runs with other difficulties such as learning disabilities (approximately 43%) and reading disorders (from 25 to 45%) [4] prevalence increases. While in adults, the prevalence increases with age to 17% at 50–54 years and may be greater than 70% after 60 years [5].

Signs and symptoms of CAPD include one or more behavioral characteristics—reading and writing difficulties, speech and language difficulties, difficulty hearing in background noise, difficulties in perceiving prosodic elements of speech as prosody, difficulty in following complex oral instructions, requesting repetitions of oral information, poor musical skills, sound localization difficulties, and others. This list is illustrative, not exhaustive, and it has to be remembered that these behavioral characteristics are not exclusive to CAPD [1, 6].

CAPD often occurs concurrently with other learning or developmental disabilities and is often associated with related cognitive, linguistic, or behavioral disorders. Sharma et al. [7] reported a high degree of comorbidity between APD and specific language and reading disorders. Individuals with autism spectrum disorder (ASD) and attention deficit hyperactivity disorder (ADHD) often have processing disorders [8], as well as dyslexia [9], and visual processing disorder [10].

The purpose of diagnosing testing is to identify presence of CAPD and delineate its characteristics and nature. Given the heterogeneity of the profiles of individuals who are referred for CAP assessment and their possible comorbidities, several auditory processing tests have been developed as tools for assessing different central auditory processing abilities. When selecting tests, the audiologist must recognize that a symptom may result from many underlying central auditory processing deficits (e.g., temporal processing, localization, spatial release of masking, performance with concurrent/degraded auditory signals), as well as language processing or cognitive problems. For that, diagnostic tests of central auditory function have been shown to be sensitive and specific for identification of CANS disorders.

The diversity of central hearing deficits supports the need for comprehensive test battery to track the various functions of the CANS. There is currently no universally accepted battery of APD tests. Currently, it is recommended that the behavioral assessment battery include non-verbal stimuli (temporal ordering, temporal resolution, and binaural interaction) and verbal stimuli (low redundancy dichotic and monaural listening). The battery should include tests representative several auditory processes as well as temporal processing, binaural separation, binaural integration, auditory closure, auditory discrimination, and sound localization [1].

Accompanying the behavioral assessment there should also be a carefully selected battery of behavioral tests with documented sensitivity and specificity. In a complementary way, there should be detailed observations of the case history and electrophysiological procedures, which together can provide a better understanding of CANS dysfunction [1, 6]. Even though (C)APD involves difficulties in the perceptual processing of auditory information in the central nervous system, electrophysiological auditory potentials reflect the neurobiologic activity that underlies that processing [6].

In individuals whose auditory processing skills are not developing normally, their auditory processing skills can improve with appropriate treatment. The principle underlying this improvement is called neuroplasticity. Neuroplasticity is the result of experience and stimulation and involves reorganization of the cortex and brainstem. Studies show that the central nervous system's plasticity allows for reorganization and re-mapping following experience (i.e., either cortical or brainstem stimulation), and that this neural modification is reflected in behavioral changes [11, 12]. Plasticity allows the CANS to accommodate and improve central auditory processing skills [13, 14], with continual practice resulting in learning that automatically leads to better listening skills.

2.1 Principles of CAPD intervention

Some principles are fundamental and should serve as guidelines for CAPD intervention. First, the intervention must be specific to the deficit, and personalized considering the patient's difficulties and strengths. The deficits should be clear from the results of the behavioral assessment, and the diagnosis should be given in terms of the original behavioral complaints.

The intervention should also be multidisciplinary, in most cases involving a variety of domains other than audiological, particularly if there are coexisting disorders. Checking whether CAPD is the primary disorder will help in specifying the focus of intervention and assist in prioritizing the different components and the order of their implementation.

While it is necessary to customize interventions for each individual, to maximize treatment effectiveness the treatment should incorporate both bottom-up and top-down approaches [1, 15–17]. A top-down approach focuses on auditory signal access and acquisition and includes direct auditory remediation strategies such as auditory training, as well as environmental modifications to increase signal clarity and improve the listening environment. Top-down treatments include training in core resources such as language, memory, and cognition along with environmental modifications and educational interventions [1, 16].

2.2 Comprehensive CAPD intervention

Intervention for CAPD should start as soon as possible after confirmation of diagnosis. It is important that the intervention is comprehensive and multidisciplinary, adding issues related to listening, academic and language, in addition to higher order processes such as attention, memory and executive control in auditory tasks, domains that are commonly affected by CAPD.

When planning an effective approach to treating CAPD, three main components should be included: (a) environmental changes, (b) compensatory strategies, and (c) direct intervention—that is, auditory training. All three areas must be addressed in any intervention plan for individuals with CAPD [1, 15, 16], regardless of the co-occurrence with other disorders or the subject's age group.

In addition to these three components, some guidelines in the area also recommend the use of auxiliary listening systems, such as FM systems, in the process of auditory processing rehabilitation. This is especially true if the diagnostic exam shows impairment in auditory closure skills, figure-background, and selective attention [6].

2.2.1 Environmental modifications

Environmental modifications aim to improve the individual's access to auditory information. This will involve increasing signal clarity and facilitating listening and learning in environments such as school, work, or social situations. Including bottom-up and top-down approaches based on acoustic aspects such as the use of assistive technology, environmental management that includes architectural interventions, removal of noise sources and consequently improvement of signal-to-noise ratios, and interventions for teachers and speakers including manner as information is transmitted and learned, highly redundant language aspects and listening and learning environments are highly recommended. The selection of modifications must be done systematically and must be based entirely on the difficulties presented by the individual and hearing deficits and the effectiveness of the implemented modifications must be continuously monitored [2].

2.2.2 Compensatory strategies

Compensatory strategies, also known as core resource training, are designed to address secondary deficits, strengthening higher-order functions, language, cognitive skills, and academic deficits often seen in individuals with CAPD [1, 6, 15]. Through these strategies, the individual with CAPD is encouraged to take responsibility for their own success in the listening and learning processes, encouraged to paraphrase instructions to clarify misunderstandings, and advanced problem-solving techniques are taught. Involving metacognitive (thinking about thinking) and metalinguistic (thinking about language) strategies that aim to provide compensatory methods to minimize deficits in functional listening, monitor your understanding, identify your difficulties, devise alternative solutions, and be an active listener rather than a passive listener [1, 5, 17].

2.2.3 Auditory training

Auditory training as related to CAPD aims to improve the function of the affected auditory process, the goal being to minimize or eliminate the alteration in auditory processing. Auditory training consists of an intensive series of challenging tasks based on the difficulties presented by the patient during the CAPD assessment [18].

Neuroplasticity is a great ally in the auditory training process. The nervous system is plastic and its capacity for reorganization and re-mapping by experience—neuronal modification—is reflected by behavior change [11, 12]. Changes in the neural substrate are facilitated by the presentation of stimuli in an organized, frequent, and intense way that progressively challenges the patient. The level of difficulty is appropriately graded and the stimuli are integrated into everyday activities. To maximize neuroplasticity, active participation of the patient in training is required. The inclusion of immediate feedback is important, as this gives positive reinforcement. Activities should be at or near the limit of the patient's ability [3].

Auditory training can be done formally or informally. The difference between the approaches is in the degree of control over the presentation of the stimuli and the environment. In formal training, stimuli are presented through an audiometer, allowing precise control of the level of stimulation and the types of stimuli (normally recorded). There needs to be control of intensity, frequency, stimulus duration, and inter-stimulus interval. Informal training is not concerned with stimulus control: stimuli are presented without the use of an audiometer and can be presented in person, without recordings. Informal training is carried out without the fixed "controls" needed for formal auditory training.

For auditory training to be effective, tasks must be presented systematically and graded by difficulty so that they are challenging and motivating without being exhausting. The level of difficulty is adjusted to allow the patient to achieve correct scores of approximately 70% but not less than 30% [19]. Training should be frequent and intense, considering the lengths of the sessions, the number of sessions, the intervals between sessions, and the timeframe over which the training will be performed [3, 5, 19]. To maximize motivation, performance gains, and generalization, the patient's active participation is necessary, and should be accompanied by immediate feedback and positive reinforcement. Variation of stimuli and tasks are key factors in successful auditory training [3]. The training programs that prompt these structural and functional changes must be done with auditory material different to those used in the diagnostic tests, which must be reserved only for evaluations [19].

Recent studies suggest that auditory training can serve as a valuable intervention tool for individuals with language deficit CAPD, learning difficulties, alterations in spatial processing, and adult subjects using hearing aids [6, 20–25].

Software programs are increasingly being used as strategies for auditory training. Computer-based auditory training (CBAT) provides age-appropriate strategies and presentations to keep the patient engaged. Some authors who examined children with CAPD [26], learning difficulties [26], and language and reading problems [26] have demonstrated benefits of this type of training for children with CAPD and associated issues.

3. Electrophysiology

Electrophysiology is the branch of neuroscience that explores the electrical activity of neurons and makes it possible to investigate how molecular and cellular processes react to a given stimulus. Neuronal communication takes place through electrical and chemical signals [27].

3.1 Hearing electrophysiology

The electrophysiology of hearing involves small electrical changes that can be collected through electrodes placed on different regions of the scalp. The responses are generated by structures located throughout the auditory pathway and their analysis allows us to understand the normal patterns existing in the processing of auditory information [28].

Electrophysiological techniques allow us to assess auditory information processing, giving us more information about the functioning of the central auditory nervous system. These assessment techniques have provided great advances in neuroaudiology—the field that studies the relationship between the ears and the brain [28]. Other researchers see the need for a whole new field of study related to cognitive auditory sciences which is able to provide information about the correlation between hearing and cognition. They emphasize that hearing disorders need to be treated in an interdisciplinary context, one which should include, depending on the case, the following professionals: speech therapist, psychologist, audiologist, and neurologist [3]. In this way, electrophysiological assessments can play an important role both in the process of assessing auditory processing and also in monitoring auditory rehabilitation programs, such as auditory training [29].

Electrophysiological assessment is a way of analyzing the central auditory nervous system both of patients who actively participate in behavioral assessments and in individuals whose responses appear to be unreliable. There is already a consensus that the assessment and monitoring of auditory processing is only complete when there is a combination of behavioral and electrophysiological methods.

Neuroplasticity is the basis of auditory training programs, and it acts on the connections between neurons and the myelination of neurons as a result of performing auditory tasks. The on-going benefits of auditory training programs can be monitored by performing electrophysiological assessments, measuring neurophysiological changes which occur in both the peripheral and central auditory nervous systems. Electrophysiological assessments are therefore a useful and effective tool in monitoring training programs.

Below are the results of some studies that correlated electrophysiology and auditory training. The results come from researchers who are engaged in studying the effects of auditory training through electrophysiology in different clinical populations.

3.2 Hearing electrophysiology and auditory training

3.2.1 Hearing in typically developed individuals

Research on neurophysiological changes resulting from auditory-perceptual learning for adults with normal hearing suggests that, although the auditory system responds to training, there is a substantial degree of variability among individuals in their ability to make use of physiological cues [30]. Training of auditory skills, even in individuals without complaints of alterations in the processing of auditory information, shows that changes take place in cognitive potentials (notably a reduction in latency of the P300 potential) after a program of auditory intervention [31].

3.2.2 Hearing and school difficulties

Learning results from the process of assimilating written and spoken language, and this process involves acoustic processing, phonemic processing, and linguistic processing. Integrated processing (acoustic, phonemic, and linguistic) must be complemented by the child's auditory and linguistic experience, which will be decisive for the learning of reading and writing. Researchers have found that the presence of learning difficulties is often associated with hearing deficits in children, and it is possible to monitor certain electrophysiological responses after auditory training. The results have shown an increase in the amplitude and a decrease in the latency of cortical potentials, although no changes were seen in brainstem responses [32]. The frequency following response (FFR) seems to be a very promising instrument to monitor patients with school difficulties, as well as to analyze the effectiveness of treatments, and it can be used as a biological marker of these changes [33, 34].

3.2.3 Hearing and CAPD

CAPD is defined as a disorder in one or more auditory skills involving sound localization and lateralization, auditory discrimination and recognition, temporal aspects, resolution, masking, integration, and temporal ordering. Kraus et al. [35] have reported altered responses in the following assessments: (a) brainstem auditory evoked potentials (ABRs) with click stimuli; (b) middle latency auditory evoked potentials (MLAEPs); and (c) N1 and P2 components of the long latency auditory evoked potential (LLAEP). Results have shown that there seems to be an impairment in auditory discrimination that can be observed in electrophysiological tests (mismatch negativity, MLAEP, and N1 and P2 components), as well as alterations in neural synchrony evidenced by alterations in the ABR that can impact temporal coding and the perception of sounds in the presence of noise.

3.2.4 Hearing and otitis media (OM)

Hearing deprivation, derived from multiple OM episodes in childhood, can compromise the normal development and maturation of the brainstem, as well as other cerebral and cortical structures. Diminished auditory signals can lead to desynchronization in the auditory cortex both for non-verbal and verbal sounds [36, 37]. Changes in auditory evoked potentials provide objective evidence that the auditory system has been modified [38]. One auditory evoked potential that seems to be more sensitive to deprivation from OM effects is the P300 cognitive potential [39]. The use of verbal stimuli when recording long latency auditory evoked potentials also seems to be very effective, providing additional information about auditory information processing [40].

3.2.5 Hearing and hearing loss

Hearing loss is a highly prevalent disability and, importantly, studies have shown a correlation between hearing loss and cognition. Typically, the use of a hearing aid is associated with an improvement in the speech perception. It has been observed that auditory training programs improve both the processing of auditory information and of cognitive information in individuals with hearing loss, especially in competitive listening environments [41]. Auditory training programs that include training which requires increased memory demand seem to improve speech perception in noise and, in the process, improve neural response time [42]. Electrophysiology can therefore be an extremely useful tool for recording these changes in neural velocity. Mismatch negativity (MMN) can also be used as an electrophysiological measure for monitoring changes resulting from auditory training, especially in the auditory rehabilitation of patients with hearing loss who use a hearing aid or cochlear implant [43].

3.2.6 Hearing and voice

The multisensory nature of music can have an impact on vocal production because it involves motor, auditory, and vocal mechanisms [44]. Hearing and voice are interrelated, so that the integrity of the auditory system is important for developing vocal behavior and maintaining vocal quality [45]. Individuals who sing in tune seem to have a particular pattern of responses in their FFR, showing lower latencies and stronger amplitudes than in individuals who sing out of tune. This shows that daily, long-term musical training can modify brain structures and improve the quality of auditory information processing [46].

4. Final considerations

Electrophysiological tests are important objective measures to verify the effectiveness of auditory training. In addition, it is important to emphasize that an electrophysiological evaluation plays an important role in predicting the gains to be expected from auditory training programs. Evaluation makes it possible to gauge whether the auditory training program should be continued, adjustments should be made, or a whole new intervention program begun. Thus, electrophysiological assessment is extremely important: it can indicate whether neural plasticity is possible (through improved synaptic efficiency and increased neural density) or measure the degree of functional plasticity (from behavioral changes brought about by training in auditory skills).

Author details

Milaine Dominici Sanfins[1,2*], Caroline Donadon[3], Piotr Henryk Skarzynski[4,5,6] and Maria Francisca Colella-Santos[7]

1 Child and Adolescent Heath Program, Faculty of Medical Sciences, State University of Campinas, Campinas, São Paulo, Brazil

2 Advanced Electrophysiology and Neuroaudiology Center, Department of Electrophysiology, São Paulo, São Paulo, Brazil

3 PhD Program in Child and Adolescent Health, State University of Campinas, Campinas, São Paulo, Brazil

4 Institute of Sensory Organs, Warsaw, Poland

5 Department of Teleaudiology and Screening, World Hearing Center, Institute of Physiology and Pathology of Hearing, Warsaw, Poland

6 Heart Failure and Cardiac Rehabilitation Department, Faculty of Medicine, Medical University of Warsaw, Warsaw, Poland

7 Associate Professor, Department of Human Development and Rehabilitation (DHDR), Faculty of Medical Sciences, State University of Campinas, Campinas, São Paulo, Brazil

*Address all correspondence to: msanfins@uol.com.br

References

[1] American Speech-Language-Hearing Association. (Central) Auditory Processing Disorders. Rockville, MD, United States: American Speech-Language-Hearing Association; 2005

[2] Bellis TJ, Anzalone AM. Intervention approaches for individuals with (central) auditory processing disorder. Contemporary Issues in Communication Science and Disorders. 2008;**35**(Fall):143-153. DOI: 10.1044/cicsd_35_F_143

[3] Chermak GD, Musiek FE. Handbook of Central Auditory Processing Disorder: Comprehensive Intervention. Vol. 2. San Diego: Plural Publishing; 2014. pp. 157-200

[4] Iliadou V, Bamiou DE, Kaprinis S, Kandylis D, Kaprinis G. Auditory processing disorders in children suspected of learning disabilities—A need for screening? International Journal of Pediatric Otorhinolaryngology. 2009;**73**(7):1029-1034. DOI: 10.1016/j.ijporl.2009.04.004

[5] Bellis TJ, Jorgensen LE. Aging of the auditory system and differential diagnosis of central auditory processing disorder in older listeners. In: Musiek F, Chermak G, editors. Handbook of Central Auditory Processing Disorder: Auditory Neuroscience and Diagnosis, Volume I, 2nd ed. 1st ed. San Diego: Plural Publishing; 2014. pp. 499-532

[6] American Academy of Audiology. Diagnosis, treatment and management of children and adults with central auditory processing disorder [Clinical Practice Guidelines]. 2010. Available from: https://audiology-web.s3.amazonaws.com/migrated/CAPD%20Guidelines%208-2010.pdf_539952af956c79.73897613.pdf

[7] Sharma M, Purdy SC, Kelly AS. Comorbidity of auditory processing, language, and reading disorders. Journal of Speech, Language, and Hearing Research. 2009;**52**(3):706-722. DOI: 10.1044/1092-4388(2008/07-0226)

[8] Schafer EC, Romine D, Musgrave E, Momin S, Huynh C. Electromagnetic versus electrical coupling of personal frequency modulation (FM) receivers to cochlear implant sound processors. Journal of the American Academy of Audiology. 2013;**24**(10):927-940

[9] Burns M. Auditory processing disorders and literacy. In: Geffner D, Ross-Swain D, editors. Auditory Processing Disorders: Assessment, Management and Treatment. 2nd ed. San Diego: Plural Publishing; 2013

[10] Dawes P, Sirimanna T, Burton M, Vanniasegaram I, Tweedy F, Bishop DVM. Temporal auditory and visual motion processing of children diagnosed with auditory processing disorder and dyslexia. Ear and Hearing. 2009;**30**(6):675-686

[11] Johnson KL, Nicol T, Zecker SG, Kraus N. Developmental plasticity in the human auditory brainstem. The Journal of Neuroscience. 2008;**28**(15):4000-4007

[12] Song JH, Skoe E, Wong PCM, Kraus N. Plasticity in the adult human auditory brainstem following short-term linguistic training. Journal of Cognitive Neuroscience. 2008;**20**(10):1892-1902

[13] Chermak G, Musiek F. Central Auditory Processing Disorders: New Perspectives. San Diego: Singular; 1997

[14] Gil-Loyzaga P. Neuroplasticity in the auditory system. Revue Laryngologie

Otologie Rhinologie (Bord). 2005; **126**(4):203-207

[15] Bellis TJ. Developing deficit-specific intervention plans for individuals with auditory processing disorders. Seminars in Hearing. 2002;**23**:287-295

[16] Bellis T. Assessment and Management of Central Auditory Processing Disorders in the Educational Setting: From Science to Practice. 2nd ed. New York: Thomson Learning; 2003

[17] Bellis TJ, Bellis JD. Central auditory processing disorders in children and adults. Handbook of Clinical Neurology. 2015;**129**:537-556. DOI: 10.1016/B978-0-444-62630-1.00030-5

[18] Weihing J, Chermak GD, Musiek FE. Auditory training for central auditory processing disorder. Seminars in Hearing. 2015;**36**(4):199-215

[19] Musiek F, Chermak G, Weihing J. Auditory training. In: Chermak G, Musiek F, editors. Handbook of Central Auditory Processing Disorder—Comprehensive Intervention. San Diego: Plural Publishing; 2014. pp. 157-200

[20] Alonso R, Schochat E. The efficacy of formal auditory training in children with (central) auditory processing disorder: Behavioral and electrophysiological evaluation. Brazilian Journal of Otorhinolaryngology. 2009;**75**(5):726-732

[21] Cibian AP, Pereira LD. Figure-background in dichotic task and their relation to skills untrained. CODAS. 2015;**27**(5):419-427

[22] Chermak GD, Musiek FE. Auditory training: Principles and approaches for remediating and managing auditory processing disorders. Seminars in Hearing. 2002;**23**:297-308

[23] Pinheiro FH, Capellini SA. Treinamento auditivo em escolares com distúrbio de aprendizagem. Pro-Fono. 2010;**22**(1):49-54

[24] Cameron S, Glyde H, Dillon H. Efficacy of the LiSN & learn auditory training software: Randomized blinded controlled study. Audiology Research. 2012;**2**(1):86-93

[25] Gil D, Iorio MCM. Formal auditory training in adult hearing aid users. Clinics. 2010;**65**(2):165-174

[26] Loo JHY, Bamiou DE, Campbell N, Luxon LM. Computer-based auditory training (CBAT): Benefits for children with language- and reading-related learning difficulties. Developmental Medicine and Child Neurology. 2010;**52**:708-717

[27] Carter M, Shieh J. Guide to Research Techniques in Neuroscience. 2nd ed. San Diego: Academic Press, Elsevier; 2015

[28] Skarzynski PH, Kolodziejak, Sanfins MD. Eletrofisiologia da Audição. In: Menezes PL, Sanfins MD, Capra D, Andrade KCL, de Frizzo ACF, editors. Manual de Eletrofisiologia e Eletroacústicas: um guia para clínicos. Ribeirão Preto: Booktoy; 2021. pp. 27-37

[29] Sanfins MD, Skarzynski PH, Colella-Santos MF. Speech-evoked brainstem response. In: Stavros H, editor. Advances in Clinical Audiology. London: IntechOpen; 2017. DOI: 10.5772/66206. Available from: www.intechopen.com/chapters/53013

[30] Tremblay K, Kraus N, McGee T. The time course of auditory perceptual learning: Neurophysiological changes during speech-sound training. Neuroreport. 1998;**9**:3557-3560

[31] Tremblay KL. Training-related changes in the brain: Evidence from

human auditory-evoked potentials. Seminars in Hearing. 2007;**28**:120-132

[32] Hayes EA, Warrier CM, Nicol TG, Zecker SG, Kraus N. Neural plasticity following auditory training in children with learning problems. Clinical Neurophysiology. 2003;**114**(4):673-684

[33] Sanfins MD, Borges LR, Ubilai T, Colella-Santos MF. Speech auditory brainstem response (speech ABR) in the differential diagnosis of scholastic difficulties. Brazilian Journal of Otorhinolaryngology. 2017;**83**(1):112-116

[34] Cordeiro FP, Weber MPVM, Quintino C, Skarzynska MB, Sanfins MD. Assessment of learning disorder using the frequency following response: Systematic review. The Journal of Health Science. 2020;**10**(3):9-18

[35] Kraus N, McGee T, Ferre J, Hoeppner JA, Carrell T, Sharma A, et al. Mismatch negativity in the neurophysiologic/behavioral evaluation of auditory processing deficits: A case study. Ear and Hearing. 1993;**14**:223-234

[36] Colella-Santos MF, Donadon C, Sanfins MD, Borges LR. Otitis media: Long-term effect on central auditory nervous system. BioMed Research International. 2019;**2019**:8930904. DOI: 10.1155/2019/8930904

[37] Sanfins MD, Borges LR, Donadon L, Hatzopoulos S, Skarzynski PH, Colella-Santos MF. Electrophysiological responses to speech stimuli in children with otitis media. The Journal of Health Science. 2017;7(4):9-19

[38] Shaffer EK. Auditory evoked potentials in children with and without otitis media. Texas Journal of Audiology and Speech Pathology. 1999;**XXIII**:10-20

[39] Borges LR, Sanfins MD, Donadon C, Tomlin D, Colella-Santos MF. Long-term effect of middle ear disease on temporal processing and P300 in two different populations of children. PLoS One. 2020;**15**(5):e0232839. DOI: 10.1371/journal.pone.0232839

[40] Sanfins MD, Donadon C, Borges LR, Skarzynski PH, Colella-Santos MF. Long-term effects of unilateral and bilateral otitis media and myringotomy on long-latency verbal and non-verbal auditory evoked potentials. International Archives of Otorhinolaryngology. 2020;**24**(4):e413-e422

[41] Ferguson MA, Henshaw H, Clark DA, Moore DR. Auditory training improves listening and cognition in complex conditions. International Journal of Audiology. 2002;**51**:220-227

[42] Anderson S, White-Schwoch T, Choi HJ, Kraus N. Training changes processing of speech cues in older adults with hearing loss. Frontiers in Systems Neuroscience. 2003;7:97. DOI: 10.3389/fnsys.2013.00097

[43] Kraus N, McGee T, Carrell T, King C, Tremblay K. Central auditory system plasticity associated with speech discrimination training. Journal of Cognitive Neuroscience. 1995;7:27-34

[44] Wolfe J, Garnier M, Smith J. Vocal tract resonances in speech, singing, and playing musical instruments. HFSP Journal. 2008;**3**(1):6-23

[45] Selleck MA, Sataloff RT. The impact of the auditory system on phonation: A review. Journal of Voice. 2014;**28**(6):688-693. DOI: 10.1016/j.jvoice.2014.03.018

[46] Sanfins MD, Gielow I, Madazio G, Honorio F, Bordin T, Skarzynska MB, et al. Frequency following response in adults who can or cannot sign in tune. The Journal of Health Science. 2020;**10**(3):58-67

Section 2

Auditory Brainstem Responses and Latency Evoked Potentials

Chapter 3

Short-Latency Evoked Potentials of the Human Auditory System

Gijsbert van Zanten, Huib Versnel, Nathan van der Stoep, Wiepke Koopmans and Alex Hoetink

Abstract

Auditory Brainstem Responses (ABR) are short-latency electric potentials from the auditory nervous system that can be evoked by presenting transient acoustic stimuli to the ear. Sources of the ABR are the auditory nerve and brainstem auditory nuclei. Clinical application of ABRs includes identification of the site of lesion in retrocochlear hearing loss, establishing functional integrity of the auditory nerve, and objective audiometry. Recording of ABR requires a measurement setup with a high-quality amplifier with adequate filtering and low skin-electrode impedance to reduce non-physiological interference. Furthermore, signal averaging and artifact rejection are essential tools for obtaining a good signal-to-noise ratio. Comparing latencies for different peaks at different stimulus intensities allows the determination of hearing threshold, location of the site of lesion, and establishment of neural integrity. Audiological assessment of infants who are referred after failing hearing screening relies on accurate estimation of hearing thresholds. Frequency-specific ABR using tone-burst stimuli is a clinically feasible method for this. Appropriate correction factors should be applied to estimate the hearing threshold from the ABR threshold. Whenever possible, obtained thresholds should be confirmed with behavioral testing. The Binaural Interaction Component of the ABR provides important information regarding binaural processing in the brainstem.

Keywords: auditory evoked potential, auditory brainstem response, ABR, click evoked ABR, frequency-specific ABR, objective audiometry

1. Introduction

Auditory Evoked Potentials (AEP) are electric potentials from the auditory nervous system that can be evoked by presenting abrupt acoustic stimuli to the ear. Registration of the electric potential as a function of time after stimulus presentation shows a reproducible pattern of waves that occur at specific time points after stimulus onset. The time between stimulus onset and occurrence of an extreme value of a wave is called latency. As can be appreciated from **Figure 1**, responses span a time window of several orders of magnitude ranging from several milliseconds to a second. This wide range can be divided into three time-windows reflecting

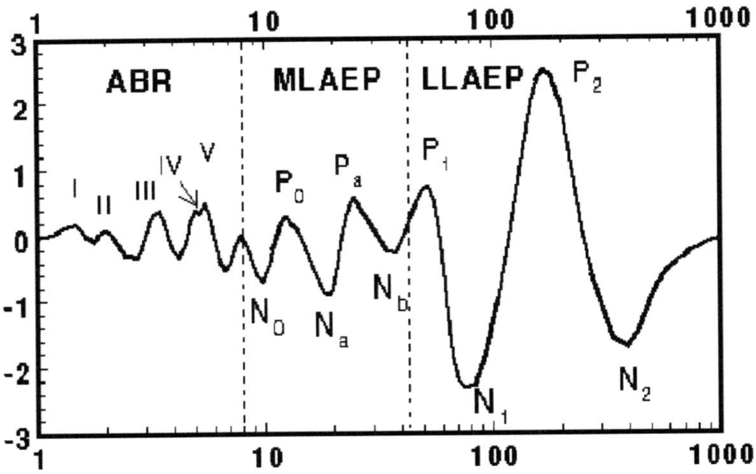

Figure 1.
Impression of registration of an auditory evoked potential. The abscissa shows latency in ms after stimulus onset on a logarithmic scale. The ordinate shows the amplitude of the electric potential in µV.

different latency ranges. Registrations within these different time-windows are generally called Auditory Brainstem Response (ABR) for short time-windows up to 8 ms, Middle Latency Auditory Evoked Potentials (MLAEP) from 8 ms up to approximately 40 ms, and Long Latency Auditory Evoked Potentials (LLAEP) for time-windows of 40 ms and longer. In this chapter we will focus on short latency ABR responses.

Figure 2 shows the results of a PubMed search with terms "auditory" and "potential" and "brain stem" and "human" (the latter both in text and as mesh term). It can be appreciated that the first paper mentioning "auditory potential" was published in 1948, but it was not until the early 1970s that the subject generated a substantial number of publication year by year. In the early 1970s, Jewett and Williston [1] introduced labeling of vertex-derived positive extremes of the ABR waves with roman numerals. They also established that these waves are far-field potentials from subcortical structures, providing indirect evidence that wave I is volume-conducted from the eight cranial nerve. Furthermore, they concluded that "waves I through VI have sufficient reliability to be worthy of establishing clinical and experimental norms". This makes them, and particularly wave V, suitable for objective audiometry based on wave occurrence and latency. Picton et al. [2] extended ABR nomenclature by introducing the prime for the vertex-negative extreme following a positive extreme. Thus V′ identifies the vertex-negative extreme following vertex-positive extreme V. In this chapter, we will refer to the vertex-positive extremes as peaks. The first intracranial recordings in humans were, to our knowledge, reported by [3, 4]. In the first study, potentials were recorded from the intracranial part of the auditory nerve in patients undergoing operations for cranial nerve disorders. The results indicated that the auditory nerve gives rise to the first two of the peaks in the scalp-recorded ABR and not to only the first peak. The latter study concluded on the basis of in-depth recordings during brain surgery that waves II and III are primarily generated within the pons, with possible contributions from the auditory nerve. Waves IV and VI originate from the pons and the medial geniculate body respectively. In Section 2 we will discuss the sources of the ABR more extensively.

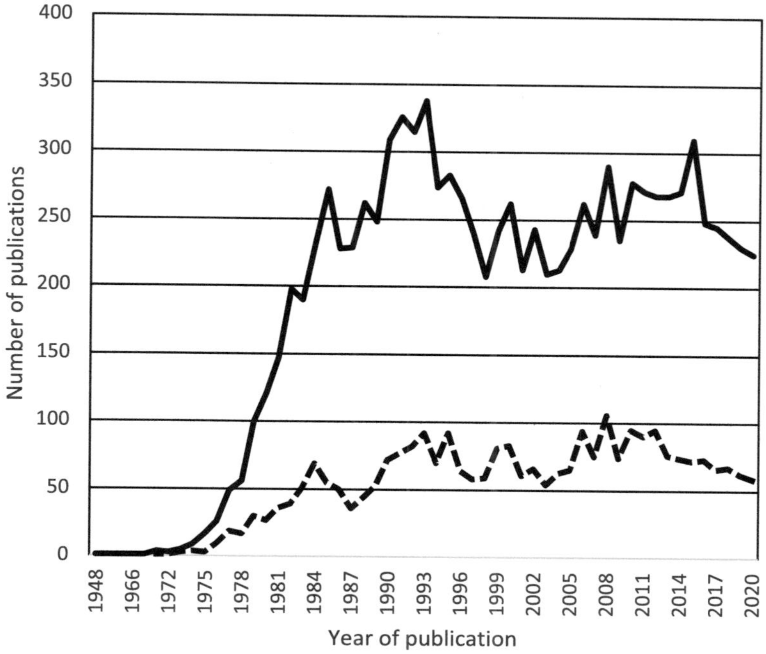

Figure 2.
Number of publications with search terms "auditory" and "potential" and "brainstem" (solid line) and "auditory" and "potential*" and "brainstem" and "audiometry" (dashed line). The term "Human" was used as a search term both in full text and as a Mesh term.*

Clinical application of ABRs includes identification of the site of lesion in retrocochlear hearing loss, establishing functional integrity of the auditory nerve, and objective audiometry. With the advent of Magnetic Resonance Imaging (MRI) for the detection of acoustic neuroma, the clinical use of ABR for this purpose has declined. ABR remains an important tool, however, for establising neural functional integrity in cases of suspected auditory neuropathy and objective audiometry in newborns. Section 3 will give an overview of all aspects of clinical ABR measurements.

Many countries have established Universal Newborn Hearing Screening Programs for the identification of children with permanent congenital hearing loss. Outcomes of these programs include a lower age of identification, lower age of provision of amplification, and better speech production and perception [5]. Infants who do not pass newborn hearing screening are referred for diagnostic audiological assessment to determine the degree and type of hearing loss, and hearing loss configuration. Hearing thresholds in newborns are typically estimated by using ABR for objective audiometry because behavioral techniques such as Visual Reinforcement Audiometry (VRA) or Conditioned Play Audiometry (CPA) are not feasible at a very young age. Another application of ABR is the detection of ototoxicity in young children that are treated with cisplatin for cancer or (concomitantly) with aminoglycosides or glycopeptides antibiotics for infections. Section 4 will discuss the application of frequency-specific stimuli for objective audiometry in these patient groups. Finally, in Section 5 we will discuss an example of the application of binaural ABR measurements as an objective measure of directional hearing ability.

2. Neural sources underlying the ABR

The structures that contribute with their stimulus-evoked electrical activity to the ABR are the auditory nerve, cochlear nucleus, superior olive complex, and the lateral lemniscus. These structures will be briefly described with respect to their physiological responses and function.

Comprehensive overviews are provided for instance in [6]. Since the ABR is often used, both in the clinic and in animal experiments, to assess hearing loss caused by damage in the cochlea, that structure is included.

2.1 Description of pathway

Sound reaches the cochlea via the outer ear canal, tympanic membrane, and middle-ear ossicles. The sensory organ in the cochlea, known as the organ of Corti, is located on the basilar membrane, which stretches from the base near the footplate of the stapes to the apex. Due to gradients of its mechanical properties from base to apex the basilar membrane functions as a frequency filter bank and it is tonotopically organized: it maximally vibrates to high frequencies of the sound at the base and to low frequencies towards the apex, and each place along the basilar membrane corresponds to a frequency it is most sensitive to, a characteristic frequency (CF). Vibrations start at the base and travel towards the apex, a phenomenon known as the traveling wave. Consequently, cochlear responses occur faster after stimulus onset to high frequencies than to low frequencies.

In the organ of Corti, two types of sensory hair cells are distinguished: inner and outer hair cells (IHCs and OHCs, respectively), which are arranged in four rows in the ratio 1:3 and which differ distinctly in function. The IHCs act as mechano-electrical transducers passing through the acoustical information to the nerve, and the OHCs act as amplifiers, increasing detection sensitivity by 40–50 dB and increasing frequency selectivity. In both types of hair cells, acoustical vibrations are converted to electrical potentials. In IHCs these receptor potentials trigger action potentials in the nerve. For that purpose, each IHC is innervated by 10–20 afferent auditory nerve fibers, which are myelinated and which systematically vary in spontaneous rate (SR) and the threshold at their CF [7], the latter allowing for a wide dynamic range to be encoded. In the OHCs, the receptor potentials trigger the cells to contract and expand, and this motility is thought to amplify the basilar membrane vibrations, in particular at low sound levels. Irrespective of the mechanisms, OHC loss leads to a threshold shift of 40–50 dB and deterioration of frequency tuning. Each OHC is innervated by a single unmyelinated afferent fiber, and it shares this fiber with several other OHCs. These fibers have very high thresholds (>90 dB SPL). The great majority of the afferent auditory nerve fibers (~95%) receive input from the IHCs. An auditory nerve of a young normal-hearing subject contains about 35.000 fibers.

Action potentials that are generated at the IHC synapse are propagated along the auditory nerve to the cochlear nucleus (CN). The nerve branches to three divisions of the nucleus: anterior ventral cochlear nucleus (AVCN), posterior ventral cochlear nucleus (PVCN), and dorsal cochlear nucleus (DCN). The AVCN contains for the large part bushy cells which show similar responsiveness as the auditory nerve fibers. Their onset response latencies are ~0.6 ms longer than that of the nerve fibers [8]. Notably, the timing of the action potentials is more precise than that of the auditory nerve, i.e., when stimuli are presented repetitively, the action potentials have a very similar latency. The PVCN contains, among other cell types, multipolar cells which show so-called chopper responses with longer latencies than the bushy cells. The frequency tuning in AVCN and PVCN is similar to that in the auditory nerve. The DCN has a complex circuitry of various cell types including inhibitory interneurons. Consequently, many DCN neurons show frequency tuning that is characterized by excitatory responses to limited frequency-sound level combinations, and inhibitory responses to a wide range of frequencies and levels.

The bushy cells in the AVCN project to the superior olivary complex (SOC), which is the first station along the auditory pathway to combine input from both ears [9]. Specifically, the spherical bushy cells send their precise phase-locked action potentials to both ipsi- and contralateral medial superior olive (MSO) and to the ipsilateral lateral superior olive (LSO); globular bushy cells project to the contralateral medial nucleus of the trapezoid body (MNTB) from where inhibitory input is delivered to the LSO. Receiving well-timed input from both ears, neurons in the MSO are tuned to interaural time differences (ITD), and receiving ipsilateral excitatory and contralateral inhibitory input LSO neurons are sensitive to interaural level differences (ILD).

The next station in the auditory brainstem is the lateral lemniscus (LL), which globally can be distinguished in a ventral nucleus (VNLL) processing monaural information and a dorsal nucleus (DNLL) processing binaural information. The VNLL receives input from the contralateral CN, and the DNLL receives input from ipsilateral MSO and bilateral LSO.

Monaural and binaural pathways from each of the above-described brainstem nuclei converge in the inferior colliculus (IC). It allows the IC to process several auditory features including basic spectrotemporal features [10] and 2-dimensional spatial information [11].

2.2 Contribution of various nuclei to ABR

The ABR waveform is commonly described as consisting of five peaks. Peaks III and V typically dominate peak II and IV, respectively, and are the ones to be best observed in daily practice in a clinic or laboratory. Peak I appears more prominently in animals than in humans, where it fades faster with decreasing stimulus level than peaks III and V (see also Section 3.6). Electrical activity from the auditory nerve and brainstem nuclei contributes to the ABR. A first-order approach to understand which neural population corresponds to which peak, is to consider the sequence of nuclei in the pathway. The inter-peak interval of approximately 1.0 ms agrees with the axonal conduction time and synaptic delay between the generation of action potentials at two successive neurons. Indeed, as summarized by [12] for the human ABR partly based on intraoperative recordings, peak I reflects the activity of the auditory nerve, peak III that of the CN, peak IV the SOC, and peak V the LL. Peak II is generated by the central part of the auditory nerve, likely where it branches to the three CN divisions. In smaller mammals used in auditory research like gerbils, mice, and guinea pigs, rather four than five peaks are distinguished with peak IV being analogous to peak V of the human ABR [12]. A fifth peak would then reflect responses in IC, as a correspondence to IC evoked potentials in mice indicated [13]. Based on a series of careful lesion and modeling studies of click-evoked ABRs in cats, [14] linked peak I to the auditory nerve, II to the globular bushy cells in AVCN, III to spherical bushy cells and cells driven by globular cells, IV to MSO principal cells, and V to cells driven by MSO principal cells.

In a secondary approach, one should consider that the early stations besides contributing to early peaks can also contribute to later peaks. We consider the ABR evoked by the most commonly used stimulus, a broadband click. As a consequence of the traveling wave mechanics, the click response latency in the auditory nerve is shortest for high-CF neurons and increases with decreasing CF [15], which leads one to conclude that high-CF fibers contribute to wave I [14]. The low-CF fibers with longer latencies and multi-peaked responses (with inter-spike intervals of 1/CF) therefore may contribute to later waves. In particular for high click levels, the high-CF fibers show second firings about 1 ms after the first action potential, an interval that is related to the neural refractoriness [16], and notably, similar to the ABR inter-peak interval. The same notion applies to the CN bushy cells, i.e. those with lower CFs have longer click latencies and may contribute to later peaks.

2.3 Summing contributions from the various sources

The following factors determine the extent to which a neural population contributes to the ABR: the number of responding neurons, the discharge probabilities of the individual neurons, the discharge latencies, the synchronization of discharges between neurons, the synchronization of the individual neuron, and the unit response (UR). How action potentials of a neural population shape an ABR wave is illustrated in **Figure 3** by the compound action potential (CAP), which reflects the auditory nerve response, thus analogous to wave I of the ABR. The CAP is mathematically described as the convolution of the compound discharge latency distribution (CDLD) and the UR, a concept introduced by [18]. An example of a CAP with corresponding CDLD and UR is shown in **Figure 3**, along with the convolution equation.

The CDLD is the sum of the discharge probabilities of all responding auditory nerve fibers, which are typically recorded by poststimulus time histograms (PSTHs) acquired by presenting the stimulus a few 100 times. The discharge probability is the ratio of discharges and the number of stimuli. The synchronization is high when to

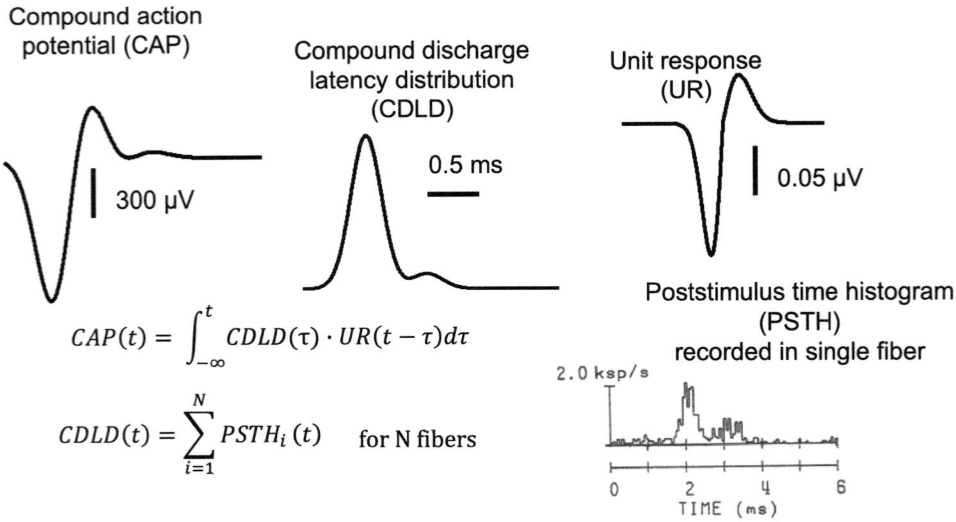

$$CAP(t) = \int_{-\infty}^{t} CDLD(\tau) \cdot UR(t-\tau)d\tau$$

$$CDLD(t) = \sum_{i=1}^{N} PSTH_i(t) \quad \text{for N fibers}$$

Figure 3.
Example of CAP and corresponding CDLD, which is constructed based on the CAP and depicted UR using the convolution equation. The UR is modeled after experimental guinea pig data [17], and the PSTH is an example of a recorded single-fiber response to 256 presentations of a monophasic condensation click of 100 μs.

each stimulus presentation the latency is very similar, thus resulting in a peaky PSTH, and the synchronization is low when the discharges are spread. The click-evoked PSTH in **Figure 3** has a latency of about 2.0 ms with some discharges at 1.8 ms and some at 2.3 ms; the second peak reflects second discharges of the neuron. The CDLD will be relatively narrow when the PSTHs of the responding neurons have the same latency, and broad when the latencies vary among neurons. The latter applies to the auditory nerve since fibers with a low SR have typically longer latency than the fibers of high SR [15]. The UR is the potential at the recording electrode that results from a single action potential. Obviously, it determines both the size and shape of the AEP waveform, and it depends mostly on the distance of the electrode from the neural population. Generally, the UR depends on specific electrode configurations, the tissue between electrode and neurons, which includes electrodes at the skin, and skull characteristics. It is the factor that is most difficult to assess; for the CAP, it has been assessed by recording the potential at the CAP-recording site around the occurrence of action potential [17, 19, 20]. Each neuron may have its UR depending on the neuron's location and morphometry. For the auditory nerve it can be assumed that the UR does not vary significantly with CF and SR [17], an assumption that generally works well when using the UR to predict CAPs [21–23]. The neural populations in the brainstem, however, will have URs that vary greatly between nuclei [14].

As an approximation, the CAP amplitude is proportional to the number of responding neurons (N in equation in **Figure 3**). **Figure 4** shows amplitudes of CAPs evoked by an electrical current pulse as a function of the number of auditory nerve fibers in guinea pigs.

Most of these guinea pigs have been deafened and consequently, the number of neurons, quantified by packing density of the cell bodies in Rosenthal's canal at different durations of deafness, varied widely [25]. Using an electrical stimulus, synchronization

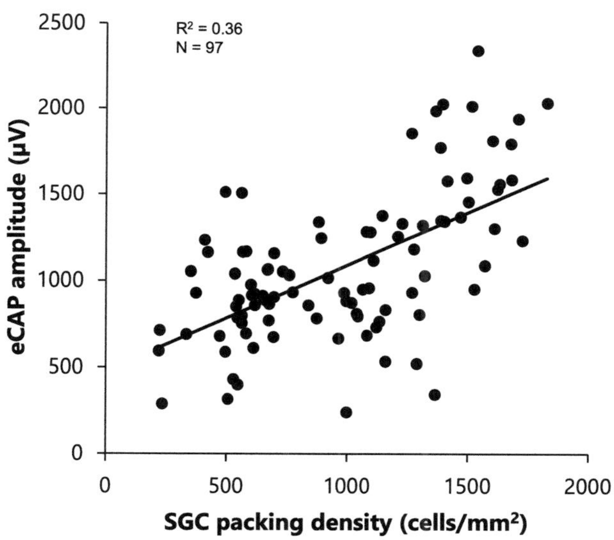

Figure 4.
Amplitudes of CAPs to electrical pulse stimulation (eCAPs) as a function of packing density of spiral ganglion cells. Data are acquired in 97 guinea pigs that are normal-hearing or ototoxically deafened with varying duration of deafness (2–14 weeks). Electrical pulses used were biphasic pulses with a phase duration of 50 µs and inter-phase gap of 30 µs and alternating polarity. Current levels are maximal, i.e., at or near saturation. The packing density reflects the number of surviving neurons. For methodological details see Ramekers et al. [24].

is expected to be large, and the great majority of surviving neurons are expected to respond, creating an ideal condition to test the convolution approximation. Indeed, the CAP amplitude significantly increases with the neural packing density, however, the amplitude varies enormously among guinea pigs, and the variance is only explained for 36% by the packing density. This outcome confirms that the number of responding neurons is an important factor, but at the same time it underscores the unreliability of amplitude as a measure of auditory evoked potentials including the ABR.

How do responses with different latencies add up? To address that question again the CAP provides a good illustration as shown in **Figure 5**.

The example shows two CAP contributions, with a ratio second/first of 0.25, and a latency difference of CDLD of 0.6 ms (left column) and 0.4 ms (right column). The difference of 0.2 ms has enormous consequences for the resulting waveforms. The left waveform shows two distinct waves (N1, P1, N2, P2) but the right waveform shows a merged P1-P2 while the N2 has vanished. It illustrates an often occurring phenomenon of ABRs that waves appear as merged components, therefore not showing the classical 5 waves.

The URs of the various brainstem nuclei are crucial for how the potentials add up. As the URs depend on recording sites, the effect of changing electrode sites is demonstrated in **Figure 6** showing click-evoked ABRs in a normal-hearing guinea pig, first with skin needles as electrodes, second with screws implanted in the skull as electrodes. For the different click levels, the waveforms show clear differences.

2.4 Effect of hearing loss

ABR waveforms vary with degree and types of hearing loss. We discuss two different types of common pathologies with respect to the consequences for the click-evoked ABR, OHC loss in basal cochlear regions, and synaptopathy.

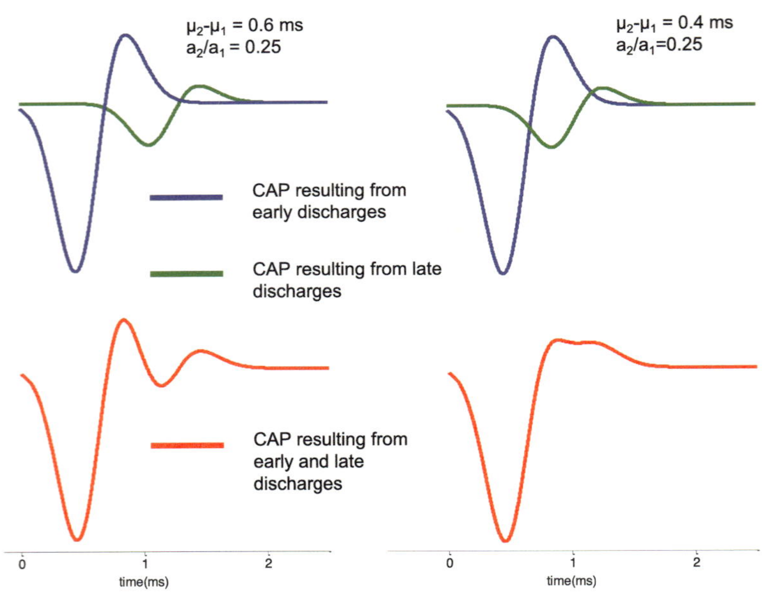

Figure 5.
Illustration of summing of two waveforms with varying latencies. In the left column, the latency difference between the first and second contribution is 0.6 ms, and in the right column, the latency difference is 0.4 ms. The size of the contributions is unchanged. The resulting waveforms (bottom row) differ greatly in that the left one shows a clear second peak, whereas the right one shows only one peak. The waveforms here show CAPs, but the principle applies to ABRs as well.

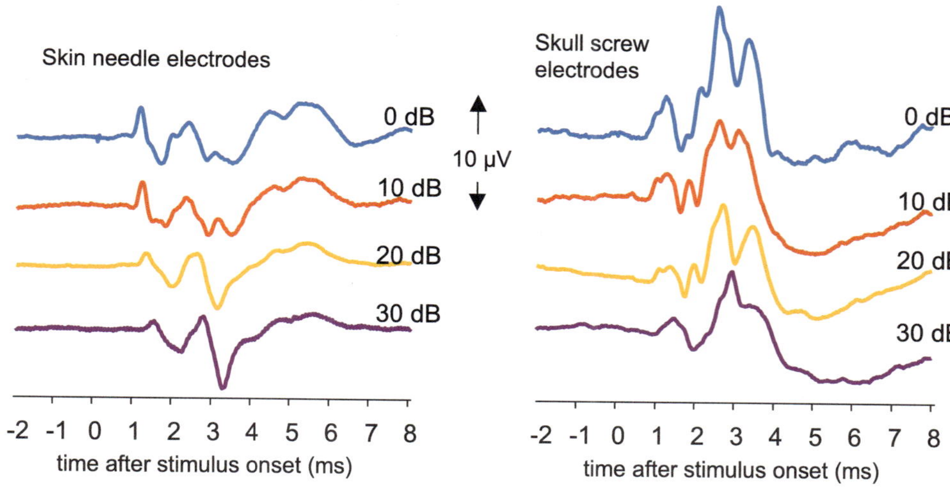

Figure 6.
Click-evoked ABRs recorded from normal-hearing guinea pigs. Clicks consisted of monophasic pulses of 20 µs with alternating polarity, presented at a rate of 10.1/s. The levels indicate dB attenuation relative to ~110 dB pe SPL. Subcutaneous needle electrode configuration: Active electrode behind the ipsilateral pinna, reference electrode on the skull, rostral to the brain, and ground electrode in the hind limb. Transcranial screw electrode configuration: active electrode 1 cm posterior to bregma, and the reference electrode 2 cm anterior to bregma; as ground electrode a subcutaneous needle electrode in the hind limb was used. For methodological details see [24].

OHC loss in basal cochlear regions, for instance, caused by ototoxic medication, noise trauma, aging, or any combination of these, leads to high-frequency hearing loss and to degradation of frequency tuning, which both have consequences for click-evoked responses of the auditory nerve. First, the latency increases with decreasing click level will be larger than normal, since for the lower levels the neurons from apical regions, which have late responses because of the traveling wave delay, will dominate the contributions to the ABR. Second, the difference in auditory nerve responses between rarefaction and condensation clicks (see Section 3.4 on stimulus polarity), which is negligible in normal ears, will increase in particular with respect to latency. Basal neurons in regions of OHC loss show decreased sensitivity for high frequencies and increased sensitivity for low frequencies [26], which can be characterized as double frequency tuning, leading to click responses with short latencies typical for high-CF click responses and latency differences between rarefaction and condensation clicks reminiscent of low-CF responses [27]. While this polarity asymmetry occurs at high click levels, at low levels the dominating low-CF responses will cause a latency difference in responses between the rarefaction and condensation polarity. Third, shallow frequency tuning may lead to increased synchronization [27], which can be explained by considering the click response as an impulse response of which the frequency tuning is the Fourier transform.

In animals, it has been demonstrated that aging leads to loss of neurons because of damage to the IHC synapses while the IHC itself remains functional [7]. Exposure to noise also when not leading to IHC loss augments this cochlear synaptopathy. The amplitude of wave I of the ABR has been found to be strongly correlated to the survival of IHC synapses in mice [28] reminiscent of the correlation between eCAP amplitude and neural survival in **Figure 4**. In humans, neural degeneration also occurs with increasing age, and speech perception has been shown to be affected by the neural loss as quantified in a post-mortem histological analysis [29]. The low-SR neurons, which have high thresholds, are especially vulnerable for synaptopathy and therefore the ratio of wave I amplitudes at high and low stimulus levels is regarded as a measure of synaptopathy. Carcagno and Plack [30] underscored the use of this ABR measure as they found a decrease in the wave I ratio with age. Alternatively, the ratio of wave I and wave V amplitudes is sometimes used.

3. Clinical ABR measurements

3.1 Recording ABRs

For clinical ABR measurements, an acoustical stimulus is presented to the patient and electrodes mounted to the skin of the head record the neural responses. Generally, short-duration stimuli are used, and the response is acquired in a time-window of about 10–20 ms starting at stimulus onset. High-quality recordings require good contact between skin and recording system. Therefore, electrodes should be applied to the skin carefully to minimize the electric impedance between electrode and skin. Many different types of electrodes are available, both disposable and non-disposable. The quality of the electrodes and their application is of utmost importance for a high ABR recording quality. Essential is that inter-electrode impedance is kept below 5 kΩ, preferably below 3 kΩ. If this cannot be achieved, then at least the interelectrode impedances should be symmetric, for instance all-around 8 kΩ, as will be explained below. Inter-electrode impedance should be kept stable during the ABR assessment, so well-fixated electrodes are required.

For single-channel ABR-recording, one electrode (the so-called active electrode) is attached to the skin, generally at the midline of the head somewhere between forehead and nape. The ABR amplitude is higher when its position is closer to the vertex. A second electrode (also called the reference electrode) is attached at ear level, for instance, close to the upper border of the mastoid plane. The position of the third (ground) electrode is not very critical. Often, an off-midline location on the forehead is chosen (see **Figure** 7), but for a single-channel recording, the ear-level position at the contralateral ear can also be used. In that case, when changing stimulation side, the reference and ground electrode should be exchanged.

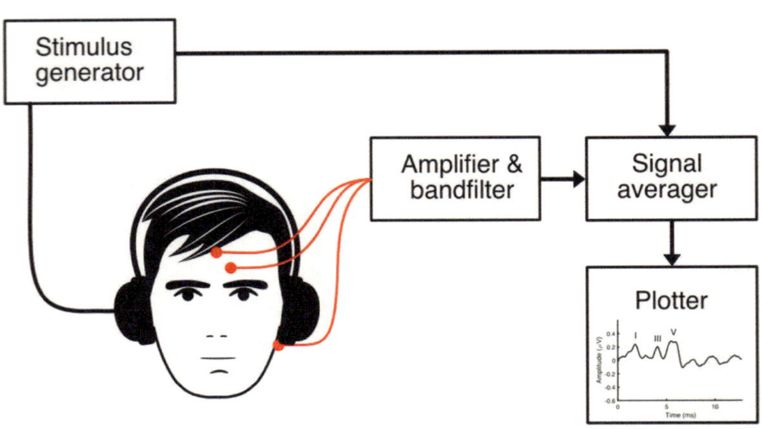

Figure 7.
Measurement setup for a single channel ABR measurement with an electrode on the midline, an electrode at ear level, and a grounding electrode off mid-line on the forehead.

ABR-potentials are also extremely small in comparison to other (interfering) potentials picked up by the electrodes. Therefore, high recording quality requires knowledge about the possible origins of these interferences and methods to reduce their strengths.

3.2 Amplifying, filtering, and averaging of the ABR signal

As ABR-potentials are in the range of 0.002–2 μV, amplification by a factor of 10,000–100,000 is required before the signals can be processed and interpreted. To achieve the high amplification factor that is required, differential amplifiers must be used. This type of amplifier has three connectors, two for input to the amplification channel (so-called plus and minus inputs) and one ground connector. Commonly, the midline (active) electrode is connected to the plus input, and the ear-level (reference) electrode is connected to the minus input. The third (ground) electrode is connected to the ground connector. In multi-channel ABR-recording systems, different channels share the active and the ground electrode. For each extra channel, only a separate reference electrode is needed. Often an ipsilateral ear-level electrode is used as a reference electrode for channel 1 and a contralateral ear-level electrode is used as a reference electrode for channel 2.

A differential amplifier suppresses the contribution of potential variations that are (approximately) common to the plus and minus input connectors, thereby reducing their contribution to the amplifier's output signal. The common-mode rejection ratio is the amplifier characteristic that reflects to what extent this suppression is successful. It should be at least 90 dB for high-quality ABR measurements. The common-mode rejection ratio degrades significantly when electrode impedances are too asymmetric, for instance, 2 kΩ for the reference electrode against 10 kΩ for the active electrode. So, inter-electrode impedance symmetry is essential for reaching a common-mode rejection ratio as high as is specified for the amplifier that is used.

Overloading the amplifier is unavoidable in ABR recording. Activation of head and neck muscles, for instance, may produce potential variations (EMG potentials) between the plus and minus connectors of 10–50 mV. To avoid overloading the first stage amplifier with an amplification factor of say 1000, the amplifier's output signal should be able to vary up to 10–50 V without saturating. Such a large output dynamic range of the amplifier requires a high power-supply voltage to avoid too many overloads. If the power supply of the amplifier cannot accommodate these high output levels, the output signal will saturate at its maximum or minimum extreme values and stay at that level for a time. Saturation generally occurs a little below the power-supply voltage. For instance, with a power supply voltage of 15 V, just below +15 V or −15 V.

One of the most important characteristics of the amplifier is its behavior when it recovers from overloads. This behavior is never listed in the specifications of the amplifier because the specifications only describe the normal functioning of the amplifier and not how it behaves after an overload. Some amplifiers show recovery behavior that makes them unfit for ABR recording, especially when the recovery potential waveform is a damped resonant. We advise to check this behavior of the amplifier, by using a single overloading pulse as the input signal.

Every ABR measurement system uses an analog bandpass filter in the input stage to suppress all non-ABR-related content of the input signal. Depending on the slopes of the passband, appropriate high pass and low pass cut-off frequencies should be selected. The steeper the slope in dB/oct, the lower the value of the high pass cut-off frequency should be. For a slope of 24 dB/oct, the high pass cut-off frequency should be as low as 10–15 Hz. A quadrupling of that range is allowed for each halving of the slope. For example, for 6 dB/oct filter slope, the high pass cut-off frequency should be set at 160–240 Hz. The low pass cut-off frequency is less critical, as long as it is above 2 kHz for a slope of 6 dB/oct, with a quadrupling per doubling of the slope. After analog-to-digital conversion that occurs at some point in the signal processing, various filter designs can be used providing such filtering uses linear phase filters. In addition to amplification and filtering, four other methods are used to suppress the interfering potentials as much as possible to improve the quality of the ABR-recording: averaging, artifact-rejection, windowing, and alternating the stimulus polarity.

Most of the interfering potentials are not synchronous with stimulus onset but start randomly at a certain time point after stimulus onset. Consequently, at a specific time-point after stimulus onset, the measured electric potential amplitude consists of the ABR amplitude (signal) at that time-point and the sum of randomly distributed interfering potential amplitudes (noise). The first component (signal) is very weak compared to the second (noise). The signal, however, is causally related to the stimulus, while the noise varies randomly in amplitude and sign. By averaging the responses of many repeated fixed-level stimulus presentations, the values of the noise potential amplitudes tend to cancel each other, resulting in an average value of zero. The average of the ABR component, however, is not zero and its relative contribution increases with the increasing number of stimulus presentations. When calculating the average value after 1000–2000 stimulus presentations, the ABR component is generally stronger than the noise component and the ABR waveform emerges from the noise. For higher ABR amplitudes, commonly at higher stimulation levels, the number of averaged single-stimulus responses can be lower than at lower stimulation levels to arrive at the same ABR signal-to-noise ratio.

Averaging the response of multiple stimulus presentations increases the signal-to-noise ratio drastically. The signal-to-noise ratio can be improved even more by a non-linear filter process called Artifact Rejection (AR). This process imposes a lower and upper limit on the electrode potential values that are accepted as valid measurements during a single registration at a fixed stimulus level. The idea is that if this value is exceeded during that registration, the response is dominated by interference and does not reflect the auditory nerve and brainstem responses. The upper and lower limit values are commonly set symmetrically as + and – a specific voltage value called the AR level. If any of the values in the sequence exceeds the AR level, the whole sequence is rejected for averaging. ABR systems in general allow the setting of the AR levels in μV, so for instance +/– 15 μV. For good quality ABR recording the AR level should be somewhere between 15 and 25 μV. Some ABR systems allow specification of the number of times that the AR levels may be exceeded before rejecting the whole sequence. For good-quality ABR recordings this number should be low, close to zero. Other signal averaging systems do not use stimulus amplitude as an AR criterion, but the AR rate. For instance, say that to have arrived at 1500 accepted responses for averaging, 1650 stimuli had to be presented. In other words, the responses to 1500 stimuli were accepted and the responses to 150 stimuli were rejected. In that case, the rejection count was 150, and the rejection rate was 150/1650. Setting an AR rate instead of absolute response amplitude levels for AR may result in accepting averages that are dominated by a few contaminated responses with high potential amplitudes, for example of myogenic origin. In terms of statistics, this approach may lead to a higher type II error probability (i.e. the mistaken acceptance of a false null hypothesis). Therefore, we advise against the use of such averaging systems for clinical ABR assessment.

In unweighted averaging, every accepted response sequence after a stimulus presentation contributes equally to the average value after say 1500 stimulus presentations. In weighted averaging, however, each accepted response sequence is assigned a weight. This weight is calculated by some paradigm. For example, the weight could be determined by one over the variance of the sequence. This results in a final average with a larger contribution of the sequences with less interference (=lower variance). Manufacturers of ABR measurement systems generally do not specify the specific paradigm used in their system. Combining weighted averaging with AR is sometimes called Bayesian AR. This procedure uses weighted averaging for stimuli that are still within specified AR limits, assigning less weight to responses with higher amplitude. Responses with amplitudes that lie outside the AR limits are still rejected.

3.3 Identifying interfering potentials

To get a grip on the always present interference, one needs to know the origins of interfering potentials. The interfering noise can be synchronous to (or in sync with) the stimulus or not. In the first case, averaging does not help to reduce the amplitude of the interfering components. Furthermore, the interfering components can be of the physiologic origin or not.

Interfering potentials with a physiologic origin are potentials generated within the patient's body, e.g. by muscles, the brain, the eyes. Muscle activations are the most powerful source. Due to the differential type of amplification, only muscles at the head cause significant interference. Their interference comes in two different kinds. (1) In sync with the stimulus, caused by the (strong) auditory stimulation used with the ABR recording. The muscles involved are located postauricular (the muscles that can move the pinna) and in the neck (the sternocleidomastoid muscle). (2) Not-in-sync with the stimulus, caused by muscle activation at the level of head and neck, with muscles of the neck and jaw as major sources. The brain is also a source of interfering potentials, albeit normally much weaker than myogenic potentials in the ABR-frequency band. All brain activity not related to the auditory system causes interfering potentials. The eye is also a weak source of interference in the ABR-frequency band.

Non-physiological interference can be introduced by the recording and stimulation system itself, by other (medical) devices coupled to the patient, and by irradiation from external sources. The ABR-system can introduce interference by (1) the auditory stimulator used for eliciting the ABR, the so-called stimulus-artifact, or (2) error or poor electrical design of the system.

Generally, the stimulator contains an electrodynamic loudspeaker that generates an electromagnetic wave resulting from its coil movements. This waveform mirrors the electrical stimulus waveform (more specifically, convolved by the stimulator's impulse response). If this coil is close to electrodes or their leads an artefactual potential variation is introduced by electromagnetic induction. Obviously, this interfering potential is in sync with the stimulus and is not reduced in strength by averaging.

The most frequent causes of error are mains interference caused by ground loops originating in the amplifier and are caused by poor design of its power supply. For instance, the power supplies of the stimulus amplifier and the physiologic amplifier should be completely independent. If not, the supply voltage of the physiologic amplifier can suffer a dip when a strong stimulus is presented. Due to the extremely high amplification factor of the physiologic amplifier, even a very small dip can cause a significant output signal variation. This may incorrectly be interpreted as input signal variation. Another example: in a multi-channel recording system the power supplies of the amplifiers of different channels should be independent and mutually completely decoupled to keep the common-mode-rejection factors independent.

Coupling of the patient to other medical equipment, like a heart-lung monitor in the intensive care unit or operation theater, often causes ground loops confounding the physiologic amplifiers' function with mains interference. The patient, the electrode wiring, and the pre-amplifier are also antennas that pick up the electromagnetic fields from the environment by induction. There is a multitude of possible sources, like radio broadcasting, wireless telephones, pagers, automatic doors, etc.

3.4 Reducing interference

Identification of the origins of the interfering signals requires inspection of the raw amplified electrode signal during the averaging process. This can be done by observing a free-running registration that is in sync with stimulus presentation.

When the difference in skin-electrode impedance is high for different electrodes (inter-electrode impedance), non-physiological interferences generate higher interfering potentials in the ABR measurement system. Therefore, keeping inter-electrode impedances below 5 kΩ and preferably below 3 kΩ, helps to reduce the interference induced by stimulus artifact and electromagnetic irradiation. If this interference is still too strong, it helps to lower the inter-electrode impedances even further down to under 1 kΩ.

The stimulus artifact has the waveform of the convolution of the electrical stimulus waveform and the stimulator's impulse response. With any waveform of the stimulus, there is first compression or reduction of the air pressure in the ear canal, the air is first condensed or first rarefied. The stimulus polarity is named accordingly: condensation or rarefaction. By alternating the electric stimulus polarity in the series of say 1500 stimuli used for one stimulation level, the alternating waveforms of the stimulus-artifact cancel each other from one stimulus to the next, because these are in anti-phase. At higher stimulation levels, however, the impulse response of the transducer might be somewhat asymmetric as to the phase, and therefore subsequent stimulus artifacts do not cancel exactly anymore. As a result, a stimulus artifact will remain present in the averaged response. This will occur specifically at levels close to the output limits of the transducer and with damaged transducers (after a drop to the floor for instance).

Increasing the number of averaged (accepted) responses increases the signal-to-noise ratio of the resulting ABR waveform. This only holds, however, for stationary noise. In clinical measurements, ABR interfering noise is in general very non-stationary in character. Therefore, averaging more than 2500 sweeps generally does not result in further improvement of the signal-to-noise ratio.

As myogenic potentials generate the strongest interference, the ABR-recording quality can be greatly improved by reducing muscle tension in the patient. This can be done by several conservative methods. (1) Placing the patient in a relaxing position in a special chair or on a bed, with special attention for a relaxed head position. (2) Keeping the patient's head position in the midline. Asymmetric pre-tension of both sternocleidomastoid muscles may lead to an asymmetric and stronger muscle-artifact in sync with the stimulation. (3) Showing a (soundless and non-thrilling) video at a height that forces the patient to steer the eyes to the midline of the lower half of the view field. When such measures do not suffice, additional (medical) measures can be taken, of course with medical authorization and/or control. (1) Giving relaxing drugs to the patient (obviously with authorized control). Some drugs, like ketamine, are unfit however because they provoke abnormal brain activity with higher interference in the ABR-frequency band as a result. (2) Giving full anesthesia with muscle relaxation and ventilation. In that case, however, care must be taken that the anesthesia is deep enough. Light anesthesia causes an enhancement in the higher-frequency components of the EEG, resulting in enhanced interference in the ABR-frequency band.

3.5 Recording strategy

To provide ABR-recordings with as much information as possible, the following procedures will help. (1) Make a two-channel recording at each stimulus level. (2) Create separate (sub)averages for different combinations of stimulus polarity, i.e. a (sub)average for condensation, rarefaction, and alternating polarity. (3) Create (sub) averages for test-retest measurements. (4) Record ABR responses at various levels of stimulation, spanning the (remaining) dynamic range of the auditory system for the side of stimulation, with five different levels if possible. (5) Present the different ABR recordings ordered vertically with the highest stimulus level on top. This creates an ABR pattern, that facilitates inspection of peak latency shift against stimulus intensity. If separate registrations for test-retest or condensation-rarefaction polarity are available, pairwise presentation per stimulus level is preferred. (6) Repeat steps 4–5 interactively during ABR assessment to arrive at the optimum result in the available time for assessment, "biding your time". This way the next stimulation level to be measured can be chosen optimally.

In two-channel recordings, the active electrode of an amplification channel is commonly positioned at the midline of the head, e.g. the vertex, and the reference electrodes at ear-level. With the reference-electrode at the side of stimulation, the ipsilateral ABR is recorded. With the reference electrode at the ear opposite to the side of stimulation, the contra-lateral ABR is recorded. The ipsi- and contralaterally measured ABR waveforms differ in specific aspects that can help to identify the ABR waveform peaks I–V. The most important differences are (1) peak III has a somewhat shorter latency in the contra-laterally derived ABR-waveform; (2) peak V has a somewhat longer latency in the contra-laterally derived ABR-waveform. With the ipsilateral recording projected right above the contralateral one in the visual representation, a kind of trapezoidal shape is visible in the peaks III–V combination. This greatly helps identifying that combination, specifically if the peak I–II combination is difficult or impossible to identify (see **Figure 8**).

The ABR waveforms for condensation and rarefaction stimulus polarities are not identical. This can only be made visible when responses for different stimulus polarities are recorded separately. A major problem with measuring the ABR responses for different stimulus polarities in different measurement runs is that due to the non-stationary nature of noise, these responses are measured under different interfering noise conditions. This can be avoided by measuring ABR responses with an alternating stimulus-polarity and storing the corresponding responses in separate data buffers. This allows creating subaverages for condensation and rarefaction stimuli that are acquired in similar noise conditions. When data of the different buffers are summed, the alternated average is still visible, but it can be split into two separate parts. Projecting the one superimposed on the other (with a different color for

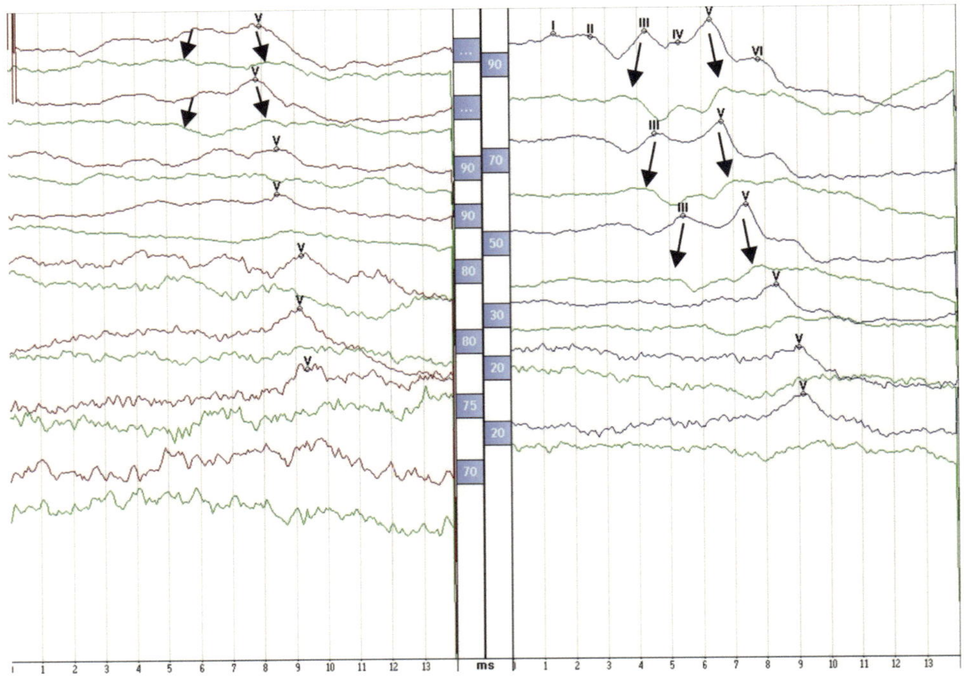

Figure 8.
Example of the simultaneous presentation of ipsi- and contralateral registration of ABR-response, showing the trapezoidal shape of the peak III–V complex.

example) makes the differences between responses from condensation and rarefaction stimulus polarities visible. One obvious difference that stands out is the form of the stimulus-artifact, which is of opposite polarity. Concomitantly, if the cochlear microphonic response is detectable within the stimulus artifact, it will also show different polarity. Major differences can also occur in the morphology of III–V peak complex in cases of (steep) high-frequency cochlear hearing loss, as was explained in Section 2.4. These differences can be so large that identification of the III–V complex is ambiguous in responses obtained with alternating stimulus polarity, while identification is straightforward in the responses obtained with condensation or rarefaction polarity separately.

Additional information can also be derived by creating separate data buffers for alternating test and retest registration to again obtain subaverages acquired in similar noise conditions. Projecting test-retest subaverages on top of each other in different colors enables quick visual inspection of the stability of the acquired ABR responses, to determine if the ABR peaks robustly rise above the residual noise floor (see **Figure 9**). This can not only be judged subjectively, but the two subaverages also allow for quantitative calculations of various measures of similarity.

In summary, sorting the single stimulus responses into four data buffers, subaveraging and making various combined or split views of the results, yields easily available information on the stability of the results and of the differences between condensation and rarefaction responses.

Preferably five or more responses for different stimulation levels are acquired to construct an ABR pattern. As measurement time is often precious, due to the requirement of the patient remaining in a relaxed condition, it is best to aim at first acquiring

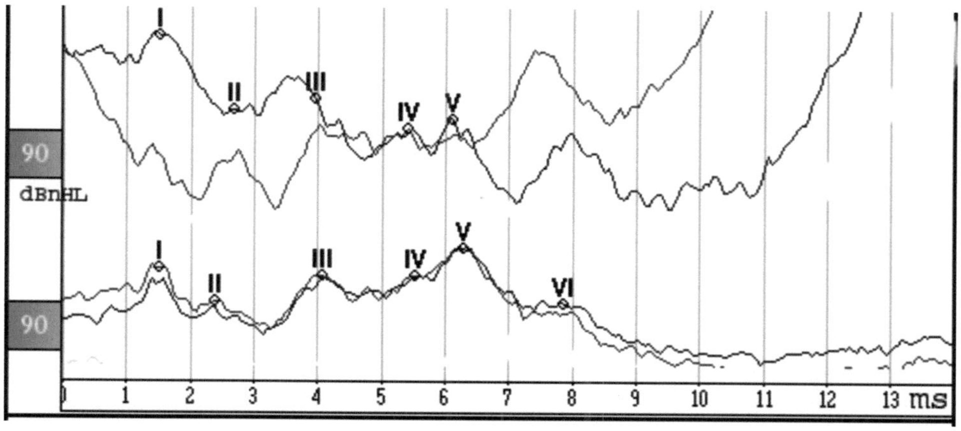

Figure 9.
An example of the presentation of test-retest subaverages. The upper registration shows a case with low test-retest reproducibility and the lower registration shows a case with high test-retest reproducibility.

ABRs at higher stimulation levels and then at levels between 25 dB above and around the response threshold. In the lower-level range, the stimulus step size should be 10 or even 5 dB, while at levels far above threshold larger step sizes of 20 or even 25 dB can be used. Each succeeding stimulation level should be chosen as time-efficiently as possible. This can be achieved by constructing the ABR pattern each time acquisition at a specific stimulus level is completed. If a succeeding acquisition with a much lower stimulus level produces no ABR response, an educated guess should be made for the next higher level to be used.

The response threshold is defined as the lowest stimulation level at which reproducible response peaks (generally peak V) can be identified. At levels up to 20 dB above threshold and 5 dB below threshold, replication measurements are advised to confirm the presence or absence of response peaks. Note that for response threshold assessment, at least one acquisition must be obtained that shows no response peaks at all, preferably at a stimulation level just below (say 5 dB below) the lowest stimulation level that shows reproducible peaks in the response. Obviously, this is not necessary if response peaks are found at levels in the normal range of the response threshold, i.e. 0–20 dB(nHL). To enable good interpretation of the results for the various stimulation levels, it is very useful to order the recordings vertically according to decreasing stimulus levels, preferably in pairs of ipsi- and contralateral responses. This way of constructing the ABR pattern enables tracking of ABR peaks from high stimulus levels down to threshold, as is demonstrated in **Figure 8**.

3.6 Interpreting ABRs

The first step in ABR pattern interpretation is peak identification. The second step in the audiological use of the ABR pattern is determining its validity, i.e. whether the ABR pattern reflects the neural integrity of the auditory nerve and brainstem. The third step is determining the response threshold level. The fourth step is analyzing the relations between latency of the peaks and stimulus level.

First, identify peaks in the ABR pattern with equal or higher latency for decreasing stimulation level. At higher stimulation levels, say above 85 dB(nHL), peak latencies may be stable, at lower stimulation levels peak latencies increase with decreasing stimulation level. Commonly this increase is larger when the stimulation level approaches the response threshold. Identification of the peak I–III–V complex is commonly easiest, and even more so with 2-channel recording with the ipsilateral averaged response positioned above the contralateral averaged response as shown in **Figure 8**. A trapezoidal shape should be observable in this complex, which positively identifies the III–V complex. Reproducibility of amplitude and latency of a peak at a constant stimulation level is required for reliable peak identification. As explained above, a test-retest view of the response pattern is very helpful. Easy switching between the views on the overall average and test-retest sub-averages helps to achieve greater reliability of peak identification.

Next, the peak I–II complex should be identified. Commonly the complex is better identifiable in the ipsilateral recording than in the contralateral recording. At high stimulation levels, over 85 dB(nHL), peak I prevails in amplitude and peak II is visible as a kind of shoulder on the downslope of peak I. At lower stimulation levels peak II tends to prevail in amplitude and peak I is visible as a kind of shoulder on the upslope of peak II. The transition range is between 55 and 65 dB(nHL) in normal hearing. Below 55 dB(nHL) peak I is rarely visible, but peak II can be. Mistakenly identifying peak II as peak I, yields an abnormally short time interval between this peak I and peak V. Identification of the I–II complex can be difficult or impossible in cases of significant conductive hearing loss. Then one must rely on the identification of the III–V complex for interpreting the ABR results.

Before performing audiometry based on the ABR pattern, the neural integrity of the auditory nerve, which is the source of the measured peak I and II potentials, should be assessed. This can be done by measuring the inter-peak interval, i.e. latency differences between peaks. For adults with normal auditory nerve function, the I–V latency difference should be below 4.3 ms. Larger differences are suspicious and the reliability of the audiometric interpretation of the pattern is questionable. These limits are age-dependent, and for patients below 2.6 years, this limit value is higher. For term-born neonates it is 5.4 ms and for preterm neonates it is still higher. However, it must be kept in mind that absolute latencies can be prolonged due to a conductive hearing loss. In that case, the effective stimulation level of the cochlea is lower than the stimulation level by the amount of conductive loss. For each type of ABR system the normative values of the absolute latencies may differ somewhat, depending on the design and the stimulator used. Therefore, the absolute latencies of peak III and V at a specific stimulation level should preferably be compared to their normal range for that type of equipment setup.

With high-quality ABR-registrations, identification of the response threshold level is easy. In the case of moderate quality, identification is still possible but requires more expertise and experience. Two independent experienced judges will generally disagree by not more than 5–10 dB. For audiometric interpretation, the correspondence between the ABR threshold and pure tone threshold depends on the type of stimulus used, i.e. tonal or broadband. In the latter case, when a click stimulus is used, for example, the ABR threshold is strongly correlated with the pure-tone audiometric threshold at 3 kHz [31] as further discussed in Section 4. The latter being 10 dB less in dB(HL) than the ABR threshold in dB(nHL). In cases of very steep cochlear high-frequency hearing loss, the difference becomes larger, because the pure-tone frequency of highest correlation with the ABR threshold shifts downward. One should be on guard for this pitfall if shallower shapes of the ABR peaks are observed. For tonal stimuli, the relations between ABR threshold and pure-tone threshold depend strongly on the stimulus waveform used for eliciting the ABR.

4. Frequency-specific ABR

This section gives a brief overview of frequency-specific ABR techniques that are now commonly used to establish hearing thresholds in audiological assessment following the newborn hearing screening and discusses why these techniques may be considered appropriate.

Traditionally, 100 μs click stimuli are used to evoke ABR responses (**Figure 10a**, top left). There are a number of advantages of using this stimulus: (1) it generally results in well-formed and detailed responses, (2) it helps in determining auditory neuropathy, and (3) it generates relatively large responses and therefore responses can be obtained in a brief amount of time [32]. Various studies describe a good correlation between click-evoked ABR thresholds and behavioral thresholds in the 2–4 kHz range, e.g. [31, 32], with correlations as high as 0.94. However, other studies report issues with the use of click stimuli for threshold estimates and report a much poorer correlation [33, 34]. The click-evoked ABR may seriously over-or underestimate sensory hearing loss, depending on hearing loss configuration. Though click ABR thresholds correlate well with the 2–4 kHz region on a population level, this does not necessarily result in accurate threshold estimates for individual patients. Stapells & Oates attribute these issues to the broadband spectrum of clicks and conclude that the click-ABR threshold probably represents the "best" hearing in a wide frequency range [33].

Over the years, several methods for obtaining frequency-specific ABR thresholds have been explored, for example, involving ipsilateral masking of frequency regions or derived response methods with filtered clicks. Hall gives a review of these various approaches [35]. The most common clinical approach for recording frequency-specific ABRs is more straightforward and involves brief tone stimuli, or tone-bursts. A tone-burst stimulus is a transient stimulus of typically 5 tone cycles within a Blackman window (**Figure 10a**), or a 2 cycles rise-time-1 cycle plateau-2 cycles fall-time envelope [35]. This stimulus configuration gives an acceptable trade-off between

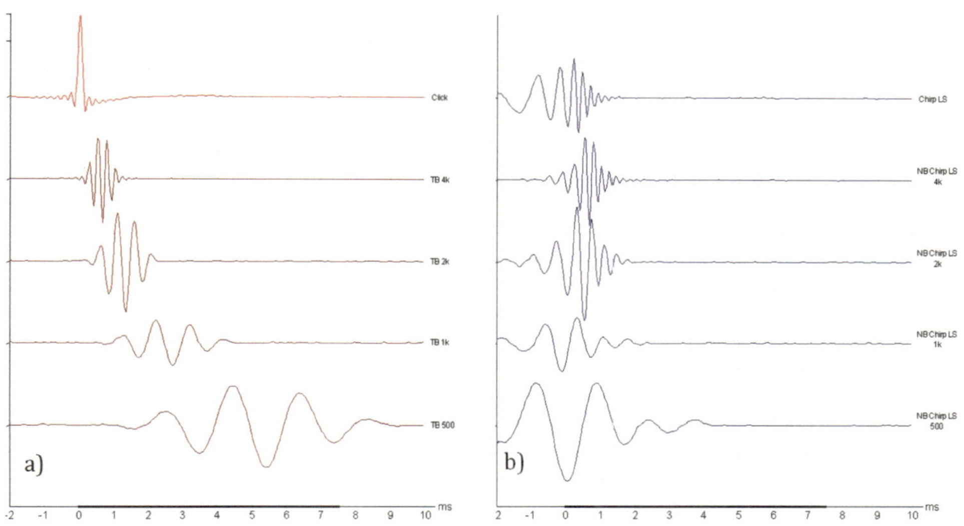

Figure 10.
Waveform of ABR stimuli as recorded with an interacoustics eclipse loopback test (a) 100 μs click, 4, 2, 1, 0.5 kHz Blackman window tone-burst stimuli (b) broadband LS-CE chirp, 4, 2, 1, 0.5 kHz NB-CE chirp.

the short stimulus onset needed to evoke an auditory response, and the bandwidth needed to obtain frequency specificity. Several studies describe high correlations (0.85–0.95) between pure tone audiometry thresholds and tone-burst ABR thresholds in adults [36, 37] and in infants [34, 38] and the authors conclude that tone-burst ABR is a clinically feasible and accurate method of estimating the pure tone audiogram when appropriate correction factors are applied.

Larger and clearer ABR responses can be evoked by using chirp stimuli, mathematically designed to compensate for frequency-dependent traveling wave delays in the cochlea and to generate synchronous stimulation across a wide frequency region. These level-specific (LS) chirp stimuli generate larger amplitude responses than clicks or tone-bursts, thus increasing the signal-to-noise ratio and reducing test time [39]. Elberling and Don derived narrow-band (LS NB-CE) chirps from these broadband chirps with approximately one-octave bandwidth (**Figure 10b**) [40]. These LS NB-CE chirps facilitate frequency-specific ABR.

Ferm et al. found significantly larger ABR responses with LS NB-CE Chirp stimuli compared to tone-bursts and anticipated a vast reduction in test time for achieving a similar SNR [41, 42]. They also established correction factors, compensating for the offset between ABR threshold (dB nHL) and estimated hearing level (dB eHL), as well as threshold confidence intervals for these stimuli. These correction factors are currently in use in the British Newborn Hearing Screening Program (Guidelines for the early audiological assessment and management of babies referred from the Newborn Hearing Screening Programme. British Society of Audiology, 2014).

5. Binaural auditory brainstem responses

An important feature of the auditory system is the ability to determine the location of sound sources relative to the head. Information from two ears can be used to estimate the location of a sound source in the horizontal plane using ITD and ILD. Using these binaural cues, normal hearing individuals can localize with high accuracy and precision [43]. Auditory localization allows humans to quickly detect and orient towards relevant sounds in the environment. This can be important, for example, when trying to safely navigate through traffic by bike or when walking, or when trying to focus on a single conversation in a noisy environment.

Measuring auditory localization accuracy and precision in a clinical setting requires specialized setups with a large number of speakers and, ideally, eye- or head-tracking. Although objective measures of hearing ability are often applied in the clinic, objective measures of auditory localization are not frequently used or well-known. An interesting objective measure of auditory localization can be found in the Binaural Interaction Component (BIC) of the ABR since the later peaks (IV and V) originate from binaural nuclei SOC and LL (see Section 2.2).

The amount of binaural interaction between the ears can be used as an objective measure of binaural hearing. ILDs and ITDs can be presented via headphones by introducing level and time differences between the left and right channels of a stereo sound. The BIC can be obtained by subtracting the ABR to a stereo sound from the sum of the monaural left and right ABRs [44, 45]. In normal-hearing listeners, the binaural ABR and the monaural sum are not the same, resulting in a different waveform: the BIC (see **Figure 11**). The most prominent peak in the BIC is the first negative peak, often called DN1 (sometimes called beta). The amplitude and latency of the DN1 systematically vary with ILD and ITD in humans and animals [46–48].

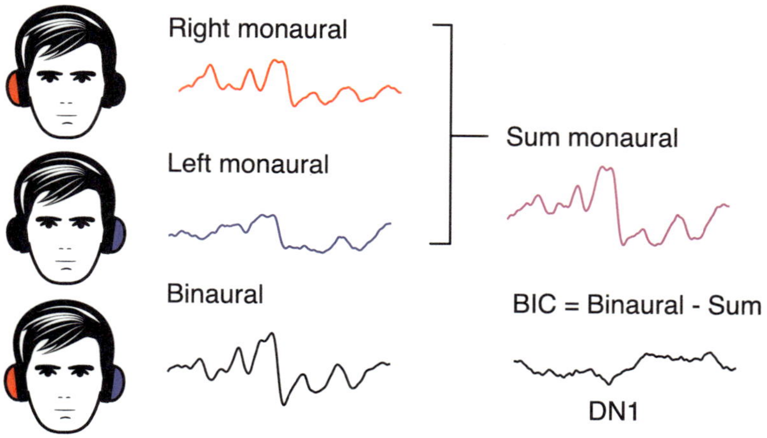

Figure 11.
The BIC is calculated by subtracting the binaural ABR from the sum of the monaural ABRs. Figure obtained from Laumen et al. [45].

The largest amount of interaction (the largest DN1 amplitude) is typically observed at an ILD of 0 dB and/or an ITD of 0 μs.

The DN1 amplitude, and thus the amount of binaural interaction, gradually decreases with increasing ILD or ITD. The most likely sources of the DN1 are the MSO and LSO in the SOC [45].

Given that the BIC is a difference waveform and the fact that ABR peaks are typically of low amplitude, measuring the BIC requires a high signal-to-noise ratio in the binaural and monaural ABRs. Additionally, to obtain the DN1 amplitude for multiple ILDs requires a quite extensive testing and may be less practical in the clinic where less time may be available for measurements [48]. Some studies also report that the BIC is absent for some participants with normal localization skills (e.g. [49, 50]), making it difficult to rely on for individual diagnostic purposes in some cases. However, the BIC can be used to study the processing of binaural cues in the brainstem in various populations at a group level. For example, a study of children at risk for central auditory processing disorders (CAPD) showed that their BIC amplitude was reduced relative to normal hearing children [51]. Interestingly, the children in the CAPD group showed normal ABR thresholds, suggesting that binaural interaction can be specifically affected in certain conditions. That the presence of the BIC has some diagnostic value can be seen in the results of a study in which the presence of the BIC was used to detect children at risk for CAPD. The investigators could distinguish between children at risk for CAPD and those not at risk with a 76% sensitivity and specificity [52].

To conclude, the BIC of the ABR provides important information regarding binaural processing in the brainstem. Although some studies suggest that it may not be the best objective measure for diagnosing binaural hearing disorders at an individual level, it does provide a unique window into binaural cue interactions early in the auditory processing pathway.

6. Conclusions

Sources of the ABR are the auditory nerve and brainstem auditory nuclei. Clinical application of ABRs includes identification of the site of lesion in retrocochlear hearing loss, establishing functional integrity of the auditory nerve and objective audiometry. To help interpretation and establish reliability, separate subaverages may be obtained for ipsi- and contralateral registrations, and for test-retest reliability. Hearing threshold estimation of infants who are referred for audiological assessment after hearing screening relies on accurate estimation of hearing thresholds. Frequency-specific ABR using tone-burst or narrow band chirp stimuli is a clinically feasible method for this. Whenever possible, obtained thresholds should be confirmed with behavioral testing. The binaural interaction component of the ABR provides important information regarding binaural processing in the brainstem. Although some studies suggest that it may not be the best objective measure for diagnosing binaural hearing disorders at an individual level, it does provide a unique window into binaural cue interactions early in the auditory processing pathway.

Author details

Gijsbert van Zanten[1,2], Huib Versnel[1,2], Nathan van der Stoep[3], Wiepke Koopmans[4] and Alex Hoetink[1,2*]

1 Department of Otorhinolaryngology and Head and Neck Surgery, University Medical Center Utrecht, Utrecht University, Utrecht, The Netherlands

2 UMC Utrecht Brain Center, Utrecht University, Utrecht, The Netherlands

3 Department of Experimental Psychology, Helmholtz Institute, Utrecht University, Utrecht, The Netherlands

4 The Dutch Foundation for the Deaf and Hard of Hearing Child, Amsterdam, The Netherlands

*Address all correspondence to: a.e.hoetink@umcutrecht.nl

References

[1] Jewett DL, Williston JS. Auditory-evoked far fields averaged from the scalp of humans. Brain. 1971;**94**(4):681-696. DOI: 10.1093/brain/94.4.681

[2] Picton TW, Hillyard SA, Krausz HI, Galambos R. Human auditory evoked potentials. I. Evaluation of components. Electroencephalography and Clinical Neurophysiology. 1974;**36**(2):179-190. DOI: 10.1016/0013-4694(74)90155-2

[3] Møller AR, Jannetta PJ. Comparison between intracranially recorded potentials from the human auditory nerve and scalp recorded auditory brainstem responses (ABR). Scandinavian Audiology. 1982;**11**(1):33-40. DOI: 10.3109/01050398209076197

[4] Hashimoto I. Auditory evoked potentials recorded directly from the human VIIIth nerve and brain stem: Origins of their fast and slow components. Electroencephalography and Clinical Neurophysiology. Supplement. 1982;**36**:305-314

[5] Yoshinaga-Itano C, Manchaiah V, Hunnicutt C. Outcomes of universal newborn screening programs: Systematic review. Journal of Clinical Medecine. 2021;**10**(13):2784. DOI: 10.3390/jcm10132784

[6] Palmer AR. Anatomy and physiology of the auditory brainstem. In: Burkard RF, Don M, Eggermont JJ, editors. Auditory Evoked Potentials: Basic Principles and Clinical Application. Baltimore: Lippincott Williams & Wilkins; 2007. pp. 200-228

[7] Kujawa SG, Liberman MC. Synaptopathy in the noise-exposed and aging cochlea: Primary neural degeneration in acquired sensorineural hearing loss. Hearing Research. 2015;**330**:191-199. DOI: 10.1016/j.heares.2015.02.009

[8] Rhode WS, Smith PH. Encoding timing and intensity in the ventral cochlear nucleus of the cat. Journal of Neurophysiology. 1986;**56**:261-286. DOI: 10.1152/jn.1986.56.2.261

[9] Yin TCT. Neural mechanisms for encoding binaural localization cues in the auditory brainstem. In: Oertel D, Fay RR, Popper AN, editors. Integrative Functions in the Mammalian Auditory Pathway. New York, Berlin, Heidelberg: Springer; 2002. pp. 99-159

[10] Versnel H, Zwiers MP, van Opstal AJ. Spectrotemporal response properties of inferior colliculus neurons in alert monkey. The Journal of Neuroscience. 2009;**29**:9725-9739. DOI: 10.1523/JNEUROSCI.5459-08.2009

[11] Zwiers MP, Versnel H, Van Opstal AJ. Involvement of monkey inferior colliculus in spatial hearing. The Journal of Neuroscience. 2004;**24**:4145-4156. DOI: 10.1523/JNEUROSCI.0199-04.2004

[12] Boettcher FA. Presbyacusis and the auditory brainstem response. Journal of Speech, Language, and Hearing Research. 2002;**45**:1249-1261. DOI: 10.1044/1092-4388(2002/100). Epub 2003/01/28

[13] Land R, Burghard A, Kral A. The contribution of inferior colliculus activity to the auditory brainstem response (ABR) in mice. Hearing Research. 2016;**341**:109-118. DOI: 10.1016/j.heares.2016.08.008

[14] Melcher JR, Kiang NY. Generators of the brainstem auditory evoked potential

in cat. III: Identified cell populations. Hearing Research. 1996;**93**:52-71. DOI: 10.1016/0378-5955(95)00200-6

[15] Versnel H, Prijs VF, Schoonhoven R. Single-fibre responses to clicks in relationship to the compound action potential in the guinea pig. Hearing Research. 1990;**46**:147-160. DOI: 10.1016/0378-5955(90)90145-f

[16] Prijs VF, Keijzer J, Versnel H, Schoonhoven R. Recovery characteristics of auditory nerve fibres in the normal and noise-damaged guinea pig cochlea. Hearing Research. 1993;**71**:190-201. DOI: 10.1016/0378-5955(93)90034-x

[17] Versnel H, Prijs VF, Schoonhoven R. Round-window recorded potential of single-fibre discharge (unit response) in normal and noise-damaged cochleas. Hearing Research. 1992;**59**:157-170. DOI: 10.1016/0378-5955(92)90112-z

[18] Versnel H, Schoonhoven R, Prijs VF. Single-fibre and whole-nerve responses to clicks as a function of sound intensity in the guinea pig. Hearing Research. 1992;**59**:138-156. DOI: 10.1016/0378-5955(92)90111-y

[19] Kiang NYS, Moxon EC, Kahn AR. The relationship of gross potentials recorded from the cochlea to single unit activity in the auditory nerve. In: Ruben RJ, Elberling C, Salomon G, editors. Electrocochleography. Baltimore: University Park Press; 1976. pp. 95-115

[20] Prijs VF. Single-unit response at the round window of the guinea pig. Hearing Research. 1986;**21**:127-133. DOI: 10.1016/0378-5955(86)90034-1

[21] Goldstein MH, Kiang NY-S. Synchrony of neural activity in electric responses evoked by transient acoustic stimuli. The Journal of the Acoustical Society of America. 1958;**30**:107-114

[22] Strahl SB, Ramekers D, Nagelkerke MMB, Schwarz KE, Spitzer P, Klis SFL, et al. Assessing the firing properties of the electrically stimulated auditory nerve using a convolution model. Advances in Experimental Medicine and Biology. 2016;**894**:143-153. DOI: 10.1007/978-3-319-25474-6_16

[23] Dong Y, Briaire JJ, Biesheuvel JD, Stronks HC, Frijns JHM. Unravelling the temporal properties of human eCAPs through an iterative deconvolution model. Hearing Research. 2020;**395**:108037. DOI: 10.1016/j.heares.2020.108037. Epub 2020/08/23

[24] Ramekers D, Versnel H, Strahl SB, Smeets EM, Klis SFL, Grolman W. Auditory-nerve responses to varied inter-phase gap and phase duration of the electric pulse stimulus as predictors for neuronal degeneration. Journal of the Association for Research in Otolaryngology. 2014;**15**:187-202. DOI: 10.1007/s10162-013-0440-x

[25] Kroon S, Ramekers D, Smeets EM, Hendriksen FG, Klis SF, Versnel H. Degeneration of auditory nerve fibers in guinea pigs with severe sensorineural hearing loss. Hearing Research. 2017;**345**:79-87. DOI: 10.1016/j.heares.2017.01.005

[26] Liberman MC, Dodds LW. Single-neuron labeling and chronic cochlear pathology. III. Stereocilia damage and alterations of threshold tuning curves. Hearing Research. 1984;**16**:55-74. DOI: 10.1016/0378-5955(84)90025-x

[27] Versnel H, Prijs VF, Schoonhoven R. Auditory-nerve fiber responses to clicks in guinea pigs with a damaged cochlea. The Journal of the Acoustical Society of America. 1997;**101**:993-1009. DOI: 10.1121/1.418057

[28] Sergeyenko Y, Lall K, Liberman MC, Kujawa SG. Age-related cochlear synaptopathy: An early-onset contributor to auditory functional decline. The Journal of Neuroscience. 2013;**33**:13686-13694. DOI: 10.1523/JNEUROSCI.1783-13.2013

[29] Wu PZ, O'Malley JT, de Gruttola V, Liberman MC. Primary neural degeneration in noise-exposed human cochleas: Correlations with outer hair cell loss and word-discrimination scores. The Journal of Neuroscience. 2021;**41**:4439-4447. DOI: 10.1523/JNEUROSCI.3238-20.2021

[30] Carcagno S, Plack CJ. Effects of age on electrophysiological measures of cochlear synaptopathy in humans. Hearing Research. 2020;**396**:108068. DOI: 10.1016/j.heares.2020.108068

[31] Van der Drift JF, Brocaar MP, Van Zanten GA. The relation between the pure-tone audiogram and the click auditory brainstem response threshold in cochlear hearing loss. Audiology. 1987;**26**(1):1-10

[32] Gorga MP, Johnson TA, Kaminski JK, Beauchaine KL, Garner CA, Neely ST. Using a combination of click- and tone burst-evoked auditory brain stem response measurements to estimate pure-tone thresholds. Ear & Hearing. 2006;**27**(1):60-74. DOI: 10.1097/01.aud.0000194511.14740.9c

[33] Stapells DR, Oates P. Estimation of the pure-tone audiogram by the auditory brainstem response: A review. Audiology & Neurotology. 1997;**2**(5):257-280. DOI: 10.1159/000259252

[34] Stevens J, Boul A, Lear S, Parker G, Ashall-Kelly K, Gratton D. Predictive value of hearing assessment by the auditory brainstem response following universal newborn hearing screening. International Journal of Audiology. 2013;**52**(7):500-506. DOI: 10.3109/14992027.2013.776180

[35] Hall JW. New Handbook of Auditory Evoked Responses. Boston: Pearson; 2007

[36] Canale A, Dagna F, Lacilla M, Piumetto E, Albera R. Relationship between pure tone audiometry and tone burst auditory brainstem response at low frequencies gated with Blackman window. European Archives of Oto-Rhino-Laryngology. 2012;**269**(3):781-785. DOI: 10.1007/s00405-011-1723-7

[37] Purdy SC, Abbas PJ. ABR thresholds to tonebursts gated with Blackman and linear windows in adults with high-frequency sensorineural hearing loss. Ear and Hearing. 2002;**23**(4):358-368

[38] Vander Werff KR, Prieve BA, Georgantas LM. Infant air and bone conduction tone burst auditory brain stem responses for classification of hearing loss and the relationship to behavioral thresholds. Ear & Hearing. 2009;**30**(3):350-368. DOI: 10.1097/AUD.0b013e31819f3145

[39] Elberling C, Don M. Auditory brainstem responses to a chirp stimulus designed from derived-band latencies in normal-hearing subjects. The Journal of the Acoustical Society of America. 2008;**124**(5):3022-3037. DOI: 10.1121/1.2990709

[40] Elberling C, Don M. A direct approach for the design of chirp stimuli used for the recording of auditory brainstem responses. The Journal of the Acoustical Society of America. 2010;**128**(5):2955-2964. DOI: 10.1121/1.3489111

[41] Ferm I, Lightfoot G, Stevens J. Comparison of ABR response amplitude, test time, and estimation of hearing

threshold using frequency specific chirp and tone pip stimuli in newborns. International Journal of Audiology. 2013;**52**(6):419-423. DOI: 10.3109/14992027.2013.769280

[42] Ferm I, Lightfoot G. Further comparisons of ABR response amplitudes, test time, and estimation of hearing threshold using frequency-specific chirp and tone pip stimuli in newborns: Findings at 0.5 and 2 kHz. International Journal of Audiology. 2015;**54**(10):745-750. DOI: 10.3109/14992027.2015.1058978

[43] Middlebrooks JC, Green DM. Sound localization by human listeners. Annual Review of Psychology. 1991;**42**:135-159. DOI: 10.1146/annurev.ps.42.020191.001031

[44] Dobie RA, Berlin CI. Binaural interaction in brainstem-evoked responses. Archives of Otolaryngology. 1979;**105**:391-398. DOI: 10.1001/archotol.1979.00790190017004

[45] Laumen G, Ferber AT, Klump GM, Tollin DJ. The physiological basis and clinical use of the binaural interaction component of the auditory brainstem response. Ear and Hearing. 2016;**37**:e276-e290. DOI: 10.1097/AUD.0000000000000301

[46] McPherson DL, Starr A. Auditory time-intensity cues in the binaural interaction component of the auditory evoked potentials. Hearing Research. 1995;**89**:162-171. DOI: 10.1016/0378-5955(95)00134-1

[47] McPherson DL, Starr A. Binaural interaction in auditory evoked potentials: Brainstem, middle- and long-latency components. Hearing Research. 1993;**66**:91-98. DOI: 10.1016/0378-5955(93)90263-z

[48] Riedel H, Kollmeier B. Auditory brain stem responses evoked by lateralized clicks: Is lateralization extracted in the human brain stem? Hearing Research. 2002;**163**:12-26. DOI: 10.1016/s0378-5955(01)00362-8

[49] Sammeth CA, Greene NT, Brown AD, Tollin DJ. Normative study of the binaural interaction component of the human auditory brainstem response as a function of interau.ral time differences. Ear and Hearing. 2020;**42**:629-643. DOI: 10.1097/AUD.0000000000000964

[50] Furst M, Bresloff I, Levine RA, Merlob PL, Attias JJ. Interaural time coincidence detectors are present at birth: Evidence from binaural interaction. Hearing Research. 2004;**187**:63-72. DOI: 10.1016/s0378-5955(03)00331-9

[51] Gopal KV, Pierel K. Binaural interaction component in children at risk for central auditory processing disorders. Scandinavian Audiology. 1999;**28**:77-84. DOI: 10.1080/010503999424798

[52] Delb W, Strauss DJ, Hohenberg G, Plinkert PK, Delb W. The binaural interaction component (BIC) in children with central auditory processing disorders (CAPD). International Journal of Audiology. 2003;**42**:401-412. DOI: 10.3109/14992020309080049

Chapter 4

Precocious Auditory Evoked Potential Recording with Free-Field Stimulus

Juan Bautista Calero del Castillo, Alberto Guillén Martínez and Francisco García Purriños

Abstract

The aim of this study is to determine the thresholds of normality in the recording of precocious auditory evoked potentials with free-field stimulation and to compare them with conventional stimulation with insertion headphones. For this purpose, we have carried out a case series study of children with normal hearing stimulated with insertion headphones, who underwent Auditory Brainstem Response (ABR) and Auditory Steady-State Response (ASSR) with free-field stimuli. Fifty-four ears with normal criteria of children between 6 months and 24 months of age were assessed. The latencies found with free-field stimulation in ABR were significantly longer than the latencies with insert earphone stimulation ($p<0.05$), and no differences were found in the inter-latencies. No significant differences were found in the thresholds of the ASSR response. We conclude that the ABR thresholds obtained in the free-field correspond to the delay due to the distance of the sound source to the eardrum and, therefore, are superimposable, being applicable to patients where it is not possible to stimulate with insert phones.

Keywords: auditory evoked potentials, ABR, ASSR, free field

1. Introduction

The subjective hearing test, although fundamental in the study of hearing loss, depends on the active collaboration of the patient and is, therefore, subject to the patient, is very difficult to carry out in young children and impossible in babies. Current methods of objective hearing screening, known as "Electrical Response Audiometry," are established by means of acoustic stimulation of the ear with insert earphones. This method does not exactly reproduce the natural stimulation of the ear that is carried out by sounds in our environment and which are usually transmitted through the air. With the new method we propose, using a loudspeaker, we transmit the stimulation of the ear in a natural way through the air and thus obtain results that more closely resemble natural hearing conditions [1].

IntechOpen

1.1 Generalities

The Electrical Response Audiometry quantifies and qualifies the activity of the auditory central nervous system, in the brainstem, in response to sound stimulation without the need for the active participation of the subject and in a harmless manner. This response is called "Auditory Brainstem Response (ABR)" and is registered as voltage fluctuations generated by the nervous system in response to an appropriate acoustic stimulus. For this registered response, it is necessary to extract from the electroencephalographic tracing the electrical activity coming exclusively from the auditory system [2]. The acquisition and recording of this potential require the auditory nerve stimulus to be synchronized and significant. The synchronization of the electrical activity requires very brief stimuli, which is why clicks or filtered clicks are used. This mechanical stimulus is converted in the organ of Corti into an electrical stimulus that travels along with the acoustic pathway to the auditory cerebral cortex [3, 4].

The better-registered response is now being obtained thanks to modifications in pacing parameters and response processing, together with advances in software and hardware that facilitate and simplify the register. The reduction in hardware size has allowed for less bulky equipment, facilitating mobility with the ability to be easily transported to the operating room and neonatology wards [1].

1.2 The sound

In acoustics, sound (from the Latin *sonitus*) is a longitudinal wave created by the vibration of objects from a sound source (any object capable of disturbing the first particle of the medium) and propagating through a medium. The medium is understood as a set of interlocked and ordered particles interacting with each other. The sound wave propagates by the interaction of the particles of the medium (mechanical waves), so it is not transmitted through a vacuum, unlike electromagnetic waves [5].

Literally, sensation is defined as "the impression that a living being receives when one of its receptor organs is stimulated." Therefore, we call the sensation produced in the organ of hearing by the vibratory movement of bodies (sound), transmitted by an elastic medium such as air, "hearing" [6].

The propagation in the air is determined as a function of temperature, humidity, and atmospheric pressure [7], this speed being 331.5 m/s at 0°C and 50% humidity at sea level [8]. Under these conditions, the speed of sound increases at a rate of 0.61 m/s for each degree of temperature. Therefore, in our environment, with a temperature of 22°C and a humidity of 50% at sea level, the speed of sound is 344.42 m/s [9].

1.2.1 Sound intensity assessment

The dB (decibel) is considered as a measure of intensity for the human ear. The scale that measures the dB has certain characteristics; it is logarithmic, non-linear, it is relative where 0 (zero) does not mean the absence of sound (sensation), and it is expressed with different reference levels.

The *intensity level* is determined by a reference. Zero dB indicates that the power intensity is equal to the reference [10].

The *sound pressure level* (SPL) indicates that the reference is the sound pressure.

The *hearing level* (HL) corresponds when the reference is the hearing level. It consists of a scale created to adapt dB SPL to dB HL because the human ear does not perceive different frequencies with the same intensity. In this way, the intensities and frequencies are adapted in an audiogram by weighting the intensity to obtain a linear graph that is easily readable visually. This scale considers differences at different frequencies so that 0 dB HL corresponds to the different frequencies in **Table 1**.

1.3 The human ear as a receiver of sound waves

Based on the principle of resonance, we hear sounds because the propagation of the wave in the air causes a displacement of the tympanic membrane. This displacement will result in mechanical transmission and amplification through the middle ear mechanisms and the displacement of the stapes plate. The stapes activates the basilar membrane that represents different elastic properties along with its length, being stiffer near the base and more elastic as it approaches the apex. Consequently, each segment of the basilar membrane is resonant at different frequencies, with high frequencies near the oval window and low frequencies at the opposite end. The organ of Corti sits on top of the basilar membrane, reproducing the movements of the basilar membrane and thus the movement of the stereocilia, resulting in electrical impulses that stimulate nerve fibers for central auditory processing. The combined action of the basilar membrane and the organ of Corti will create a spectral analysis, temporal identification, and intensity variation of the received sound wave which, transmitted through the acoustic pathway to the auditory areas of the cerebral cortex [11], will, in turn, create patterns of frequency, intensity and time, a fundamental process for decoding the communicative content of sound waves [5].

The human ear is an extraordinary receiver capable of receiving waves of very low intensity and can withstand, without being damaged, sounds a billion times more intense than its threshold of perception [1].

1.4 Electrophysiological basis of auditory examination

The auditory evoked potentials correspond to the recording, from surface electrodes, of the electrical activity of the acoustic pathway at the moment of an adapted sound stimulus. Therefore, to study this signal, it must be isolated from noise, that is unwanted electrical activities, such as electroencephalogram (EEG), electrocardiogram (ECG), and electromyogram (EMG), and the signal-to-noise ratio must be improved [12]. The electrical synchronization of these fibers requires very short stimuli, as in continuous noise, the unitary activity of the cochlear root is not synchronous [13].

dB SPL	Frequency in Hz
47	125
26.5	250
13.5	500
7.5	1000
11	2000
10.5	4000
13	8000

Table 1.
Correlation between dB SPL and dB HL.

From the generation of the stimulus to the activation of the cerebral cortex, approximately 300 ms elapse, a period we call "latency" [14]. However, each level of the acoustic pathway will generate a response with a different latency, which is why auditory evoked potentials will be classified according to the time segment in which we study this latency [13]. Thus:

- *Cochlear microphonic:* Corresponds to the electrical activity of the cochlea and its latency is zero.

- *Electrocochleography*: latency of 1–4 ms.

- *Auditory Brainstem Response (ABR) and Auditory Steady-State Response (ASSR)*: These are early auditory potentials with a latency of 2–12 ms.

- *Mid-latency auditory evoked potentials*: With latencies of 20–50 ms.

- *Long latency auditory evoked potentials*: With latencies of 50–300 ms.

- We focus on auditory brainstem potentials, which are considered to be early auditory potentials.

- The Auditory Brainstem Response (ABR) corresponds to the recording of the evoked response in the first 12 ms of the acoustic pathway and, almost 50 years after their discovery, they constitute one of the pillars in the study of hearing and the diagnosis of infantile hearing loss. The response is formed by a curve with 5–7 waves, the first five of which are perfectly defined and practically constant and are denominated by Roman numerals, I, II, III, IV, and V, with I, III, and V standing out as the most evident and constant (**Figure 1**) [14].

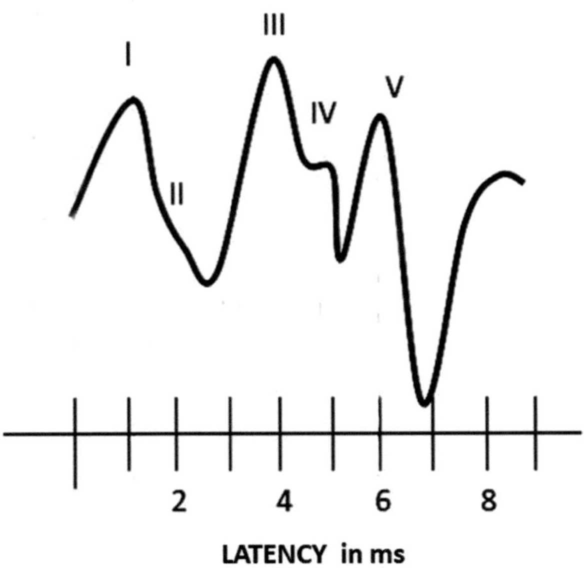

Figure 1.
Auditory brainstem response (ABR) recording.

The origin of these different waves is not clearly defined considering the complexity of the auditory pathway and the number of synaptic steps involved in its functioning [15]. However, the location of generation of each of the responses that give rise to each of the waves has been widely agreed since the 1996 studies by Melcher et al. in the cat [16]. These are as follows [5, 17–21]:

- *Wave I*: very close to the cochlea, at the level of the spiral ganglion and cochlear nerve (VIII cranial nerve).
- *Wave II*: Proximal part of the VIII cranial nerve and cochlear nucleus.
- *Wave III*: Superior olivary complex.
- *Wave IV*: Lateral lemniscus and part of the superior olivary complex.
- *Wave V*: Lateral lemniscus, inferior coniculum, and quadrigeminal tubercle.

1.4.1 Characteristics of auditory brainstem response (ABR)

Presence of response: Obviously we have to obtain the described curve with the presence of the five fundamental waves or, at least, of the three most frequent (I, III, and V) [21].

Latency: Each wave has a latency defined under normal conditions and corresponds to the time elapsed between the production of the stimulus and the appearance of the wave. Waves III and V are the most stable waves and wave I appears only at medium and high intensities [12]. The last wave in disappearing is the V-wave considering the psychoacoustic threshold at the last intensity at which its presence is observed. This threshold corresponds to frequencies between 2000 and 5000 Hz with the use of filtered clicks [22]. The interlatencies correspond to values between waves, the most important being the I-III interlatency, the III-V interlatency, and, above all, the I-V interlatency [14].

The auditory evoked potentials can already be performed at birth. From the first studies, an increased latency of wave V and a different morphology of the birth response curve have already been observed. The interlatency I-III and III-V are also increased, but to a lesser extent than I-V [23]. These changes recover progressively with age, with amplitudes at 3 months and latencies at 1 year equaling those of adults [24].

Some authors have described the latencies of neonates [17, 20], expressed in ms (**Table 2**).

Increased wave I latency is interpreted as incomplete maturation of the basal cochlear zone and/or transmission of hair cells and auditory nerve fibers. An increase in the interval of interlatency, and especially I-V, is considered to be incomplete myelination of axons and increased synaptogenesis [10].

Amplitude: The height of each wave manifests the amplitude measured in microV, although their values are very unstable.

In ABRs, a transient potential is elicited in response to a click, which returns to its initial resting state because each stimulus is followed by a sufficiently long interval before the next stimulus. But if we perform the stimulus with a sufficiently fast stimulation frequency so that the response to one stimulus is not extinguished before the emission of the next stimulus, we obtain a succession of overlapping responses. The sum of these potentials results in a sinusoidal response that will have exactly the same frequency

Pediatric ABR normative values [17, 20]				
Age	Latency MSEC			
	I	III	V	I-V
33 weeks preterm	2.57–0.54	5.68–0.75	8.21–0.79	5.64–0.70
36 weeks preterm	2.41–0.38	5.35–0.49	7.83–0.59	5.43–0.55
40 weeks term	2.00–0.31	4.82–0.44	7.14–0.43 (8)	5.14–0.40 (5.94)
40 weeks preterm	2.34–0.44	5.07–0.60	7.54–0.62	5.20–0.60
3 weeks term	1.80–0.24	4.50–0.46	6.93–0.37	5.13–0.36
3 weeks preterm	2.01–0.24	4.70–0.37	7.07–0.23	5.07–0.33
6 weeks	1.80–0.20	4.40–0.30	6.60–0.30	4.90–0.30
12 weeks (3 m)	1.70–0.20(2.1)	4.30–0.30(4.9)	6.40–0.30(7)	4.70–0.30(5.7)
26 weeks (6 m)	1.70–0.20	4.10–0.30(4.7)	6.20–0.30(6.8)	4.60(0.30)5.2
52 weeks (1 year)	1.70–0.20	4.00–0.30(4.6)	6.00–0.30(6.6)	4.30–0.20(4.7)
2 years	1.70–0.20	3.80–0.20	5.70,0.20	4.00–0.20

Table 2.
Normal values in pediatrics. Auditory brainstem response with 70 dB stimulus, with stimulation by insert earphones.

as the modulation frequency of the stimulus. These are called Auditory Steady-State Response (ASSR). Unlike transient potentials, this response will be maintained over time, as will the stimulus that provokes it [25]. Therefore, a repetitive sound at frequencies between 3 and 300 Hz evokes a steady-state response and can be said to be quasi-sinusoidal periodic responses whose amplitude and phase are maintained over time [26].

With a fast stimulation frequency range of 70–110 Hz, the overlapping transient responses are of shorter latency and generated in the brainstem similar to those of the ABR [27]. This is why they are not affected by sleep or sedation, being optimal in the study of auditory function in infants and young children [7], being this range the one used in the stimulus of our exploration.

To shorten scanning times without appreciable loss of diagnostic accuracy [25], we use multifrequency as a method of stimulating ASSRs that allows simultaneous stimulation of several frequencies, and even binaurally, requires that each tone is modulated at an identifying frequency different from the stimulation frequencies of the rest of the tones so that it can be identified later in the frequency analysis of the response [8]. We can separate in each ear the response for each frequency by evaluating the spectral component for each stimulus. In this way, we simultaneously stimulate four frequencies (500, 1000, 2000, and 4000 Hz) and both ears (ASSR-MF) [28].

To establish hearing thresholds in infants and young children, we use ABR and ASSR-MF recordings together using either insertion headphone or bone conduction stimulation, however, we are not aware of normality criteria using the free field as the sound stimulus in ABR and ASSR, that is using a loudspeaker close to the patient, a stimulus more similar to natural hearing stimulation.

The aim of this study is to determine criteria for normality in ABR and ASSR recordings with free-field stimulus and to be able to apply these neurophysiological tests in patients where they cannot be performed conventionally.

2. Material and method

We conducted a descriptive observational study of a set of cases of children aged 6–24 months from our ENT clinic at the University Hospital Santa Lucía, Cartagena (Murcia, Spain) in the period between April 2016 and January 2017 who underwent ABR and ASSR-MF using insertion earphones and ABR and ASSR-MF using free-field stimulation.

The selected patients fulfilled the criteria of normality with insertion earphones, that is with latencies and amplitudes within normality in ABR with V-wave threshold at 20 dB HL and with stabilization of responses in ASSR before 6 minutes and threshold of 20 dB HL at the four frequencies of 500, 1000, 2000, and 4000 Hz. These patients, after testing with insertion headphones, were tested again with a free-field stimulus. Children outside the age range and children with some degree of hearing impairment were excluded.

Following these criteria, the children were selected and the ABR and ASSR-MF with free-field stimulus were recorded after the conventional tests with insertion headphones, in the same exploratory act, under the same conditions, using the same sound stimulus, unilateral clicks for the ABR and amplitude-modulated tones in ASSR-MF, and taking advantage of the child's sedation. All cases were performed and recorded in the same environmental conditions, same acoustic booth, same equipment, and same explorer.

To carry out free-field stimulation, new software and hardware had to be incorporated. These modifications were carried out by the company Audiología, S.L. (Gijón, Spain), Interacoustic's technical service and distributors, and with the brand's permission. The modification of the software consisted of the possibility of choosing the use of loudspeakers in the stimulation menu, in this case using Phonestra © preamplified free-field loudspeakers whose potentiometer was mechanically fixed to avoid changing the gain of the tests.

The calibration of hearing thresholds with the correction coefficients of insert earphones is governed by IEC-60645-7 "Instruments for the measurement of auditory brainstem responses" [29]. We are not aware of any specific standards and correction coefficients for the realization of ABR and ASSR tests in the free field. For the calculation of correction coefficients, we based ourselves on the ISO-389 standard for the "zero" reference calculation in the calibration of audiometric equipment. Free-field pure-tone control audiometry was performed on 25 healthy individuals aged 14–38 years. An ASSR measurement was made in each subject, stimulating in a free field, with 0 dB correction. New correction coefficients for ASSR in the free field were obtained by the difference of the values recorded with the free-field tonal tests and the ASSR without correction, calculating a correction coefficient of 5 dB HL (±1.5 dB HL) in the four frequencies with respect to the correction rates with insertion headphones. The theoretical calculation was made following the "law of spherical divergence" by means of the behavior of sound in the free field which allows us to define the attenuation or variation of level between two previously defined points, r1 and r2 (RE: 1, 2). With these modifications and with the sound source (loudspeaker) 70 cm away from the ear to be tested, we performed the ABR and ASSR with free-field stimulus in the same environmental conditions, same booth, same equipment, and same explorer as with insertion headphones to control non-differential errors.

The tests were carried out in the rather quiet outpatient room, inside a booth with an acoustic attenuation of 38 dB SPL on average, which also houses the laptop and the explorer who operates the equipment.

The patient should be relaxed to reduce electrical noise as much as possible [30], with physiological sleep or, as in most of our cases, with mild sedation which we achieve with the oral administration of Chloral Hydrate at a dose of 75 mg/kg/weight which allows 2–3 hours of sedation. Chloral hydrate has very few adverse reactions and although it has a bad taste, it is well tolerated by children. The maximum dose of 2 g should not be exceeded and it cannot be used to maintain prolonged sedation due to the sedative effect of its metabolites [31].

After careful cleaning of the skin with alcohol, we use an abrasive cream to peel off light desquamation to reduce the resistance of the skin in the location of the electrodes that are placed once the child is asleep, placing the active electrode in the vertex, the reference electrode in the mastoid (right and left) and zygomatic region. After placing the electrodes, the ABR3A type earphones are inserted into the external auditory canal, held in place by a silicone cushion to hold them in place and to stagnate them in the size best suited to the canal orifice.

2.1 Recording the ABR with insert earphones

We stimulated with alternating clicks at a rate of 44/s with contralateral white noise masking with −30 dB HL of the stimulus intensity, using a 100 Hz high-pass filter and a 1500 Hz low-pass filter, a maximum of 4000 stimuli, a 12 ms screen window, admitting a curve quality response of 99% and a residual noise of 40 nV. The procedure is programmed using 70, 60, 40, and 20 dB HL in descending order, and the intensity can be changed manually. When it ends in one ear, it automatically starts the stimulus in the contralateral ear and we can stop the test when we consider it convenient when we have reached the threshold of wave V. In case of absence of response or poor quality of the response at 70 dB HL, we will continue with stimuli at 80, 90 or 100 dB HL until we find a graph of sufficient quality to observe amplitudes and latencies.

Once the graphs are obtained, latencies and interlatencies are measured and the results are stored for later evaluation.

2.2 Recording ASSR with insert earphones

We performed multi-frequency stimuli allowing us to stimulate both ears simultaneously at frequencies of 500, 1000, 2000, and 4000 with CE-Chirp© [17], the stimulation rate at 90 Hz, and a rejection level of 40 nV. The maximum stabilization time of the response was set at 6 minutes. We also stored the results.

2.3 Recording of the ABR with free-field stimulus

The procedure is similar to the ABR recording with insertion earphones and is carried out after performing the tests with insertion earphones and without modifying the conditions, in the same clinical act and with the patient being selected following the inclusion and exclusion criteria, as described above. Using a stimulus through a loudspeaker, selecting in the transducer menu, placed 70 cm from the ear to be tested, with masking of contralateral white noise and storing results.

2.4 Recording of ASSR with free field stimulus

Following a similar procedure to the ASSR with insertion earphones and with the modifications described for the free field, we record the ASSR with free-field stimulus after the ABR in the free field and store the results.

3. Results

Applying the inclusion and exclusion criteria, 54 ears of 27 selected children were studied, with a mean age of 16.7 months (SD = 5.7) and age range between 6 and 24 months, corresponding to 19 males (70.4%) and 8 females (29.6%).

Table 3 presents the latencies of waves I, III, and V (the most constant) and I-V interlatencies obtained with insertion headphone and free-field stimuli, as well as the differences between them. No significant differences were observed in the interlatency values.

We found statistically significant differences in the latency values of waves I, III, and V, $p < 0.001$, and Rho values of 0.78, 0.49, and 0.63, respectively. In the assessment of agreement or concordance in the distribution of mean latencies, a significant difference ($p < 0.001$) was observed in the Wilcoxon test for the three main waves of the ABR.

The V-wave threshold was obtained at 20 dB HL in all ears studied.

Table 4 represents the results of the thresholds obtained in the ASSR-MF recording with insertion headphone stimulus and in free field.

Waves	Wave I	Wave III	Wave V	Interval I-V
Insertion earphones	1.56 (SD = 0.22)	4.09 (SD = 0.29)	6.27 (SD = 0.19)	4.68 (SD = 0.46)
Free field	3.47 (SD = 0.59)	5.97 (SD = 0.61)	8.22 (SD = 0.51)	4.75 (SD = 0.36)
Difference	1.91	1.88	1.95	0.07
p	<0.001	<0.001	<0.001	
Rho	0.78	0.49	0.63	

SD: standard deviation; p: significance level; Spearman's Rho: Spearman's Rho.

Table 3.
Latencies of waves I, III and V and I-V interlatencies obtained with a stimulus with insertion headphones and free field, at 70 dB HL, as well as the differences between them, p-value and rho value in between them, p-value and rho value in Spearmen's contrast test.

Frequencies	500	1000	2000	4000
Insertion earphones	10	14	14	15
Free field	22	24	25	25
Difference	12	10	11	10

Table 4.
Results of the thresholds obtained in the ASSR-MF recording with insert earphone stimulus and in free field and the differences between the two limits (dB HL).

In the recordings with insert earphones, the 500 Hz recording was achieved in 50 of the 54 ears studied (7.41%), with responses obtained at all other frequencies. The average response stabilization time was 2.12 minutes.

In the recordings with free-field stimulus, the absence of response at 500 Hz was 22.22%, at 1000 Hz 12.96%, at 2000 Hz 5.55%, and at 4000 Hz 1.85%. The mean response stabilization time was 3.68 minutes which is an increase of 1.56 minutes over the insert phones.

4. Discussion

The children in our study are aged between 6 and 24 months, some of them premature, so latency values may be variable. This is why we decided to apply this age range to minimize variations in latencies due to the immaturity and hypomyelination of the acoustic pathway, which maturity does not end until 12 months [18, 29].

The ABR and ASSR are usually recorded by means of earphones inserted inside the external auditory canal and using surface electrodes placed as described above. The recordings of both tests taken together will give us the hearing thresholds in intensity and frequency, which are necessary for a correct objective diagnosis of hearing loss in children.

The ABR recording is composed of a 5 to 7-wave trace, with the first five waves being the most important, called I, II, III, IV, and V and I, III, and V being the most constant [15, 16] waves that present fundamental characteristics of amplitude and latency [12, 15, 23]. The latencies generate interlatencies, time intervals between waves, the most important being interlatency I-III, III-V, and above all I-V [19, 23].

These waves disappear as the intensity of the stimulus decreases, with the V wave remaining constant, the last recording of which in intensity does not mark the threshold of the response. The average values that we have obtained in the children with normal criteria studied, using acoustic stimuli through insertion headphones, are similar to those observed in the literature [17, 20, 21, 29, 32].

Likewise, the ABR study was carried out in a similar way to that employed by other authors, using the same type of stimulus (click) [33], with a cadence of 44 stimuli/sec, lower than the critical rate of 50 st/sec [34], 2000 stimuli in monaural stimulation and with contralateral masking [35].

After stimulation and stable ASSR response, the software of the device applies the Fast Fourier Transform (FFT) algorithm, which is the recording of the electro-encephalographic trace corresponding to the modulated frequency of the presented tone, and calculates the estimated audiometry at frequencies of 500, 1000, 2000, and 4000 Hz, so the normality criteria do not require detailed interpretation [10, 36] and therefore do not require the patient's cooperation or the explorer's intervention [37].

Although it is generally accepted that a stable ASSR response should not occur beyond 8–10 minutes, in our daily practice, and depending on the individual patient, we have come to accept response stabilization times of 12–14 minutes. However, in our study, we have selected cases with response stabilization of not more than 6 minutes.

We agree with the various authors that the most difficult response to record in the ASSR is the frequency of 500 Hz, with all other frequencies being fairly constant and with no differences between the two ears [10, 36, 38].

In the ASSR test, the child is in the same environment, with the same electrodes and their location on the skin as in the ABR test and with stimulation through insert earphones, the only difference being acoustic stimulation with clicks in the case of ABR and CE-Chirp in the case of ASSR. This difference does not affect the attainment of hearing thresholds, although the CE-Chirp follows a response with higher amplitude and curve quality [39].

The threshold of ASSR responses compared to hearing screening methods, such as tone audiometry or behavioral audiometry, in children has been studied by numerous authors, indicating, with minor adjustments for correction, the similarity of hearing thresholds [37, 38, 40, 41]. In our daily practice, we have found this similarity between threshold levels in older children undergoing tonal audiometry and ABR/ASSR-MF under sedation [42].

As we have already mentioned, to avoid bias, the ABR/ASSR-MF tests of the selected children, in free field (loudspeaker 70 cm away from the ear to be tested), were carried out in the same clinical act, in the same environment (cabin with acoustic attenuation), by the same explorer as in the tests with insertion earphones, first performing the stimulus with insertion earphones and then, if the child was selected, the stimulus in free field.

The performance of the tests with stimulus in the free field required the modification of the software and hardware of the equipment and its calibration, and we are not aware of any standard or correction coefficient for the performance of these tests in the free field, adjusting ourselves to the calibration performed by the company Audiología, S.L. [43].

The differences in the mean evoked latency of the ABR recording in the tests performed with insertion earphones and those in free field with 70 dB HL stimulation are presented in **Table 3**. We can see that the mean difference in the latency of the main waves (I, III, and V) corresponds to the delay caused by the distance at which the sound source is located (70 cm) in the free-field stimulation. In the conditions in which the test was performed, with an ambient temperature of 22°C, a humidity of 50%, and the cabin being located at sea level (Cartagena, Spain), the speed at which sound is transmitted in the air is 244.4 m/sec [9]. At this distance of 70 cm, the average delay of the arrival of the stimulus at the eardrum (receiver) from the loudspeaker (transmitter) is 2.032 ms, a delay that resembles the average difference of the latencies of the three waves I, III, and V of the ABR response tracing, taking into account possible variations of a few centimeters when placing the loudspeaker in each of the tests or due to the movements of the child's head during the exploration.

Likewise, the interlatencies were similar in both tests, with no significant differences between them, especially in the most important interlatency I-V, interlatencies not affected by the distance of the sound source and which shows the response of the different levels of neural generators at the level of the brainstem.

The ASSR-MF thresholds obtained with a stimulus with insert earphones in our daily practice and the selected cases are similar to those found in the literature [44–47], accepting normal values close to 30 dB HL, although there is a slight decrease in those obtained in free field in relation to those obtained with insert earphones, representing a difference of 10.37 dB HL. In our study, the mean response stabilization time was less than 6 minutes, with the most inconsistent response at 500 Hz, in both different stimulations, and the most constant responses at 1000, 2000, and 4000 Hz.

In the literature, we have found very few studies in which free-field stimulation has been used to obtain ABR and ASSR.

Shemesh et al. carried out a study with 20 patients aged between 24 and 60 years, 10 of whom underwent ASSR recording with insertion headphones, and another 10 patients with hearing aids underwent ASSR recording with free-field stimulus, comparing the thresholds. In this work, there are hardly any indications of the calibration of the equipment, although it uses a booth with acoustic attenuation according to the ISO392-2, 1994 standard. He also recorded the ASSR with and without hearing aids, finding, logically, significant differences in the thresholds with and without hearing aids, but not, on the other hand, between the thresholds with audiometry and ASSR without hearing aids. A control group of 21–24-year-olds with normal hearing recorded audiometric thresholds below 20 dB HL at frequencies between 250 and 8000 Hz and thresholds below 20 dB in ASSR at frequencies of 500, 1000, 2000, and 4000 Hz. They conclude the benefits of ASSR testing on hearing thresholds for objective assessment of the benefit of hearing aids and that it may be determinant in young uncooperative individuals [48].

Arias et al. conducted a study with 14 patients aged 2–14 years with cochlear implants to obtain ASSR-MF thresholds and behavioral audiometry. They used an Audix V, model NDOO1A USB from Neuronic, S, A., calibrated with a sound level meter model 2260 and a microphone type 4144 (Brüel & Kjaer) ensuring that the acoustic energy measured in dB SPL corresponded to its value in dB HL, but no further details are given. They did not record ABR and compared the results of ASSR thresholds with free-field stimuli with behavioral audiometry. However, the study does not give data on distance from the sound source and does not show normality thresholds as these are patients with cochlear implants and therefore profound hearing loss. They conclude that ASSR-MF recording with the free-field stimulus is useful for assessing free-field hearing thresholds in cochlear implant patients [49].

Though clinically useful, the results obtained in these studies are not comparable with those obtained in our studies since none of them examines thresholds of normality in children.

Given that there are no standards or correction coefficients for the ABR and ASSR-MF tests with free-air stimuli and the absence of sufficient literature on studies with free-field stimuli for recording early auditory evoked potentials, we consider our results as a new possibility as a determination of criteria for normality in children in whom stimulation through earphone insertion in the external auditory canal is impossible, such as children with hearing aids or implants and in those who do not cooperate in liminal or behavioral audiometry tests, such as children with down syndrome and autistic spectrum disorders.

5. Conclusions

The results obtained in this study support the usefulness of free-field stimulation as an objective method for acquiring normality criteria in ABR and ASSR tests, allowing these tests to be performed in patients who cannot be stimulated through the external auditory canal with insertion earphones, such as children with hearing aids or implantable hearing aids.

The modification of the software and hardware of the equipment currently on the market is necessary to obtain ABR and ASSR-MF recordings with free-field stimulation. The thresholds of the recordings obtained with free-field stimulation are superimposable to the thresholds obtained with current conventional insert earphones.

6. Limitations and future lines of research

The method used for the collection of auditory pathway information as a measurement instrument is widely validated worldwide.

Among possible random errors, we must take into account the variability of the measurements. We cannot control the child's head movements, even when asleep, by varying the exact distance to the loudspeaker. To minimize sampling variability, we assess the effect of chance by conducting hypothesis test.

To avoid selection bias errors, patients with perfect normal conditions with insertion earphones were selected in order to know which children without pathology could be tested with free-field stimulus.

When comparing tests performed with insert earphones and in the free field, an information bias may occur during the measurement. To avoid this bias as much as possible, we have performed the tests with the same explorer, in the same environmental conditions, with the same equipment, the same data collection, and the same processing.

Finally, there is no confounding bias as we do not want to know a cause-effect relationship in our research.

Future research should be directed toward its application in daily clinical practice with hearing-impaired children, assessing that the responses obtained with free-field stimuli are similar to the ABR/ASSR-MF values in cases of hearing pathology.

We consider the need for free-field stimulus studies in the fitting and follow-up of assistive listening devices, both conventional hearing aids and implantable devices.

Conflict of interest

The authors declare the absence of interests between the manufacturer of the equipment used (Interacoustics), the staff of the company that carried out the calibration of the equipment, and the working environment (Audiología, S.L.), or any other natural or legal person. Likewise, this work has been financed exclusively by its authors.

Author details

Juan Bautista Calero del Castillo*, Alberto Guillén Martínez
and Francisco García Purriños
Universidad Católica de Murcia (UCAM), Cartagena (Murcia), España

*Address all correspondence to: juancalerodelcastillo@gmail.com

References

[1] Calero JB. Criterios de normalidad en potenciales evocados auditivos de tronco cerebral (ABR) y potenciales evocados auditivos de estado estable (ASSR) con estímulo en campo libre [Tesis]. Universidad Católica de Murcia (España); 2019

[2] Calero JB, Guillén A, y García-Purriños, F. Búsqueda de criterios de normalidad de potenciales evocados auditivos de tronco cerebral y potenciales evocados auditivos de estado estable con estímulo en campo libre. Acta Otorrinolaringológica Española. 2019;**70**(5):258-264

[3] Biacabe B, Mon T, Avan P, Bonfils P. Anatomie fonctionnelle des voies auditives. Encycl Méd Chir, E-20-022-A-10. París: Ed. Scientífiques el Médicales Elservier SAS; 2000

[4] Calero JB, Garcillan A, y Ruano, V. Nuestra experiencia sobre el diagnóstico de las hipoacusias infantiles mediante el uso de potenciales evocados auditivos de tronco cerebral. Acta Otorrinolaringológica Española. 1982;**33**(1-2):466-471

[5] Teixeira, A, Vaz, F y Bastos, C. Física del sonido aplicada a la audición. En Manrique, M Marco, J. Audiología. Madrid: Proyectos Editoriales, S.A. 2014. pp. 43-58

[6] Real Academia Española. Diccionario de la lengua española. 23.ª ed. Madrid: Espasa; 2014

[7] Rickards FW, Lesley ET, Cohen LT, Wilson OJ, Drew JH, Clarck GM. Auditory steady-state evoked potential in newborns. British Journal of Audiology. 1994;**28**:327-337

[8] John MS, Lins OG, Boucher BL, Picton TW. Multiple auditory steady-state responses (MASTER): Stimulus and recording parameters. Audiology. 1998;**37**(2):59-82

[9] Goez Sánchez Relación de la velocidad del sonido y la temperatura. Trabajo Final. Análisis de Muestras [Internet]. 2008. Disponible en: https://es.scribd.com/doc/14690335/RELACION-DE-LA-VELOCIDAD-DEL-SONIDO-Y-LA-TEMPERATURA. Consultado: 22/10/2017

[10] Martinez Fernández A. Comparación del umbral auditivo obtenido mediante potenciales evocados de estado estable, audiometría tonal liminar y potenciales de tronco cerebral. Granada: Editorial de la Universidad de Granada; 2005

[11] Brugge JF. Patterns of organization in auditory cortex. Journal of the Acoustical Society of America. 1985;**78**(1):353-359

[12] Shomer, H. Estrategia para el registro de los potenciales evocados sensoriales (auditivos). En: Bogacz, J. Los potenciales Evocados en el Hombre. Buenos Aire (Argentina): El Ateneo. 1985, pp. 17-33

[13] Davis H. Principles of electric response audiometry. The Annals of Otology, Rhinology, and Laryngology. 1976;**85**(Suppl 2.8):1-96

[14] Trinidad GT, Trinidad G, De la Cruz E. Potenciales Evocados Auditivos. Anales de Pediatría Continuada. 2008;**6**(5):296-301

[15] Sainz, M. Potenciales Evocados Auditivos de Tronco Cerebral. En Manrique, M, Marco, J. Audiología. Madrid: Proyectos Editoriales, S.A. 2014, 147-158

[16] Bogacz J, Cols. Los Potenciales Evocados en el Hombre. Buenos Aires: Ed. Ateneo; 1985. pp. 42-68

[17] Rivera S, y Marcotti, A. Comparación de las amplitudes y latencias de la onda V del potencial evocado auditivo de tronco cerebral obtenidas a través de estímulos clic y CE-Chirp. Revista de Otorrinolaringología y Cirugía de Cabeza y Cuello. 2016;**76**:272-279

[18] Ribeiro FM, Carballo RM, Marcoux AM. Auditory steady-state evoked responses for preterm and term neonates. Audiology and Neurotology. 2010;**15**:97-110

[19] Barajas JJ. La vía auditiva dentro de tronco cerebral. Estudio anatómico funcional. In: Barajas JJ, Mencheta EM, Sainz M. Potenciales Evocados Auditivos. Madrid: Industrias Gráficas España, S.L; 1983. pp. 95-105

[20] Guilhoto LM, Quintal VS, da Costa MTZ. Brainstem auditory evoked response in normal term neonates. Arquivos de Neuro-Psiquiatria. 2003;**61**(4):1-5

[21] Norrix LW, Trepanier S, Atlas M, Kim D. The auditory brainstem response: Latencies obtained in children while under general Anesthesia. Journal of the American Academy of Audiology. 2012;**23**(1):57-63

[22] Bonfils P, Van Den Abbeele T, Ané P, Avan P. Exploration Fonctionnelle Auditive. Encycl Méd Chir, Oto-Rhino-Laryngologie. Paris: Editions Scientifiques et Médicales Elsevier SAS; 1998. pp. 20-175-A-10

[23] Barajas JJ. Potenciales Evocados Auditivos del tronco Cerebral. Descripción y características normales de la respuesta. In: Ciges M, Artieda J, Sáinz M. Stingl de Méndez M. Potenciales Evocados Somatosensoriales, Visuales y Auditivos. Albolote (Granada): Gráficas Anel, S.A; 1992. pp. 421-440

[24] Jiang ZD, Wu YY, Zheng WS, Sun DK, Feng LY, Liu XY. The effect of click rate on latency and interpeak interval of the brain-stem auditory evoked potentials in children from birth to 6 years. Clinical Neurophysiology. 1991;**80**(1):60-64

[25] Martínez-Benito, P., García, Latorre, E. Potenciales Evocados Auditivos de Estado Estable: En Manrique, M Marco, J. Audiología. Madrid: Proyectos Editoriales, S.A. 2014. p. 147-158.

[26] Pérez Abalo MC, Torres A, Savio G, Eimil E. Los potenciales evocados auditivos de estado estable a múltiples frecuencias y su valor en la evaluación objetiva de la audición. Auditio: Rev Electr Audiol. 2003;**2**:42-50

[27] Korzack P, Smart J, Delgado R, Strobel TM, Bradford C. Auditory steady-state responses. Journal of the American Academy of Audiology. 2012;**23**:146-170

[28] Lins OG, y Picton, T.W. Auditory steady-state responses to multiple simultaneous stimuli. Electroencephalography and Clinical Neurophysiology. 1995;**96**(5):420-432

[29] Salesa E. Detección precoz auditiva en neonatos. Revista de Logopedia, Foniatría y Audiología. 2008;**228**:135-137

[30] Campo M, Albiñana MS, Ferrari JM, y Herreros de Tejada, A. Utilización del Hidrato de Cloral en pediatría. Usos clínicos, preparaciones galénicas y experiencia en un hospital. Farmacia Hospitalaria. 1999;**23**(3):170-175

[31] Bickford RG, Jacobson JL, Cody DT. Nature of average evoked potentials to sound and other stimuli in man. Annals of the New York Academy of Sciences. 1964;**8**(112):204-223

[32] Wu FW, Chang H, Lin HC. Using click-evoked auditory brainstem

response thresholds in infants to estimate the corresponding pure-tone audiometry thresholds in children referred from UNHS RSS. International Journal of Pediatric Otorhinolaryngology. 2017;**95**(1):57-62

[33] Peters JF, y Squires K. Introducción a las técnicas del potencial evocado. En: Bogacz, J. Los potenciales Evocados en el Hombre. Buenos Aire (Argentina): El Ateneo. 1985. p. 1-16

[34] Beagley HA, Sheldrake JB. Differences in brainstem responses latency with age and sex. British Journal of Audiology. 1978;**12**:69-77

[35] Sainz M. Principios generales de estimulación y registro de potenciales evocados auditivos. En: Ciges M, Artieda J, Sáinz M. y Stingl de Méndez M. Potenciales Evocados Somatosensoriales, Visuales y Auditivos. Albolote (Granada): Gráficas Anel, S.A. 1992. p. 363-386

[36] Werner LA, Folsom RC, Mancl LR. The relationship between auditory brainstem response latencies and behavioral thresholds in normal hearing infants and adults. Hearing Research. 1994;**77**(1-2):88-98

[37] Pérez Abalo MC, Torres A, Savio G, Eimil E. Los potenciales evocados auditivos de estado estable a múltiples frecuencias y su valor en la evaluación objetiva de la audición. Auditio: Rev Electr Audiol. 2003;**2**:42-50

[38] Rodrigues GRI, Lewis DR. Establishing auditory steady-state response thresholds to narrow-band CE-chirps in full-term neonates. International Journal of Pediatric Otorhinolaryngology. 2014;**78**:238-243

[39] Elberling C, Don M, Cebulla M, Stürzebecher E. Auditory steady-state responses to chirp stimuli based on cochlear traveling wave delay. The Journal of the Acoustical Society of America. 2007;**122**(5):2772-2785

[40] Goldie WD. The brainstem auditory evoked potential in infants and children. The Clinical Neuropsychologist. 1992;**9**(3):934-407

[41] Stroebel D, Swanepoel De W, Groenewald E. Aided auditory steady-state responses in infants. International Journal of Audiology. 2007;**46**(6):287-292

[42] Guillén AJ, Calero JB, Martínez I. y García-Purriños, F. Correlación del umbral de potencial evocado auditivo de tronco cerebral con el umbral de potencial evocado auditivo de estado estable en pacientes hipoacúsicos. Revista de Otorrinolaringología y Cirugía de Cabeza y Cuello 2019;**79**:299-306

[43] Suárez Bascarán L. Informe de calibración de equipo de potenciales auditivos de estado estable en campo libre. S.L. Gijón – España: Audiología; 2017

[44] Françoise MN, Teissier N, Barthod G, Nasra Y. Sedation for children 2 to 5 years of age undergoing auditory brainstem and auditory steady state responses recordings. International Journal of Audiology. 2012;**51**:282-286

[45] Martínez- Benito P, Morant A, Pitarch MI, Garcia FJ, y Marco, J. Potenciales evocados auditivos de estado estable a multifrecuencia como técnica de determinación de umbrales auditivos. Acta Otorrinolaringológica Española. 2002;**53**:707-717

[46] Van Maanen A, Stapells DR. Normal multiple auditory steady-state response thresholds to air-conduction stimuli in infants. Journal of the American Academy of Audiology. 2009;**20**:196-207

[47] Rance G, Roper R, Symons L, Moody LJ, Poulis C, Dourlay M, et al. Hearing threshold estimation in infants using auditory steady-state responses. Journal of the American Academy of Audiology. 2005;**16**(5):291-300

[48] Shemesh R, Attias J, Magdoub H, Nageris BI. Prediction of aided and unaided audiograms using sound-field auditory steady-state responses. International Journal of Audiology. 2012;**51**:746-753

[49] Arias P, Hernández MC, Zuluaga P, y Calero P. Método de Evaluación en campo libre de los umbrales en pacientes con Implante Coclear: utilidad de los potenciales evocados auditivos de estado estable para la valoración del rendimiento Objetivo de los Implantes cocleares. Auditio: Rev Electr Audiol. 2015;**4**(2): 47-52

Chapter 5

Auditory Brainstem Response with Cognitive Interference in Normal and Autism Spectrum Disorder Children - Understanding the Auditory Sensory Gating Mechanism

Ahmad Aidil Arafat Dzulkarnain, Nur Hafizah Sulaiman, Fatin Amira Shahrudin, Shahrul Na'im Sidek, Hazlina Md. Yusof and Madihah Khalid

Abstract

Earlier studies disputed the influence of higher-order function such as attention or cognitive inhibition on the auditory brainstem response (ABR) result. In short, the ABR result was considered similar with or without the subject paying attention. However, in the last few years, there has been growing evidence that the higher-order function may influence the ABR findings provided the sensory gating system of the brain is triggered by any cognitive interference activities. This chapter will explain the concept of auditory sensory gating, a method to measure auditory sensory gating, and at the end of the chapter, preliminary findings concerning the ABR with cognitive interference among ten normally developing children are presented. This chapter will also share a case study that compared auditory sensory gating capacity in normal and children with mild autism spectrum disorder (ASD).

Keywords: auditory brainstem response, auditory sensory gating, Stroop task, cognitive interference, autism

1. Introduction

The auditory system through corticofugal projections connects the auditory cortex to the lower structures at the brainstem such as cochlear nucleus, inferior colliculus, and superior olivary complex [1, 2]. The auditory corticofugal system refers to the descending efferent pathway that arises from the auditory cortex. This efferent pathway plays an important role for the auditory cortex to control certain functions of the brainstem. Structures at the higher and lower brainstem on the other hand are the neural generators for the auditory brainstem response (ABR), which is one of the auditory evoked potentials (AEP) [3, 4]. Sensory gating has been reported as one of the sensory processing mechanisms generated from the corticofugal pathway [5, 6]. Since the sensory gating mechanism is known to cross this corticofugal pathway, it was hypothesized that the sensory gating processing may therefore affect the neural activity at the brainstem region and perhaps could affect the ABRs findings [1].

2. Sensory gating

The ability to filter irrelevant and repetitive stimuli and to focus only on one specific task is called sensory gating [7, 8]. Sensory gating is important to prevent sensory overload, in which individuals need to divide their attention to multiple sensory stimulations at the same time. This sensory gating response reflects the filtering function of the brain and plays a critical role as a protective mechanism of brain function. The sensory gating response through the neural inhibition mechanism prevents excessive irrelevant stimuli and sensory overload from being processed by higher brain structures. Through this process, the brain is able to process all the important information and relevant stimuli efficiently [8].

2.1 Auditory sensory gating

While sensory gating is a generic terminology that covers all sensory modalities, the auditory sensory gating is referred to as an ability of the human brain to filter unwanted or repeatable auditory input to avoid sensory overload. With optimum auditory sensory gating abilities, a human is able to focus on the target auditory signal while the other unwanted sound will remain as a background [9]. This will help individuals to listen and focus especially when they are in an environment with high background noise.

According to Jones et al. [9], auditory sensory gating is related to some of the cognitive mechanisms, namely latent inhibition and attentional inhibition, and therefore it is related to a specific-target goal set by the brain and control by the attention. A deficit in auditory sensory gating leads to abnormal sensory processing and this typically happens in children with certain disorders, for example, attention deficit hyperactivity disorder (ADHD) [10], autism spectrum disorder (ASD) [11, 12], and those with poor mental health conditions such as schizophrenia [13].

3. Assessment for auditory sensory gating

Auditory sensory gating can be measured using a perceptual scale questionnaire, behavioral psychological assessment, and auditory evoked potentials (AEP) assessments. Some examples of perceptual scale questionnaires to measure some component of sensory gating are the sensory gating inventory (SGI) [7] or structured interview for assessing perceptual anomalies (SIAPA) [14]. These scales consist of items that describe daily situations of an individual that cover their sensory processing activities involving all the sensory modalities including those from the auditory system. Individuals are asked to rate the item in the questionnaire according to the Likert scale if the situation of the sensory processing activities is relevant or not relevant to them. Recently, the sensory gating scale has been adapted for children as a parental-perceptual questionnaire in the Malay language [15].

The second method to measure auditory sensory gating is by using a cognitive interference test that is normally classified as a psychological assessment. This assessment requires individuals to do certain tasks behaviorally pertaining to the sensory gating. One of the examples of cognitive interference tests that can indirectly measure sensory gating is the Stroop task [16]. In the Stroop task, a cognitive interference effect can be elicited using color matching [17] or counting-digit techniques [18]. In Stroop counting-digit techniques, series of single digits numbers are presented repeatedly (number 4, presented as "4" or "444" or "444") to the study participants. These number series are further divided into congruent or incongruent, and additional neutral characters. Congruent number series consists of the number that is equivalent to the frequency of that number in the series (number four (4) presented four times (4444)). Incongruent number series consists of the number that is not similar with the frequency of that number in the series (number four (4) presented one time 4). For neutral series, it consists of a character that has no meaning related to the presented number (#presented four times (####). In the Stroop task assessment, patients need to indicate the frequency of the congruent, incongruent, or neutral number by ignoring the actual number or character itself. For example, for the incongruent series of *444*, the patient needs to indicate to the assessor that the frequency of the number is three instead of the number itself as four. This incongruence number series is thought to produce cognitive interference that leads to a longer reaction time for the patient to do the task and to trigger a higher number of incorrect answers in comparison to the congruence or neutral number series [19].

The third method to measure auditory sensory gating is by using auditory evoked potentials (AEP) tests. AEP is an objective measure of the auditory system neural activity in response to acoustic stimulation [20]. In standard AEP (also called obligatory AEP), the patient does not need to do anything, except relax. Recording electrodes are placed around their scalp. The recording electrodes pick up the brain's electrical activity, following acoustic or sound stimulation. The most common AEP to measure auditory sensory gating is the P1 or often called P50 component [21]. Most recently, auditory brainstem response (ABR) has been used as well to measure auditory sensory gating but with the conditions that the ABR needs to be conducted while the subject is performing certain psychological assessments (example; Stroop task) [19, 22, 23]. Both assessments are discussed in the next section.

3.1 Electrophysiology test: P50

Auditory sensory gating is well known to be recorded using the AEP test, in specific, the P50 auditory sensory gating test [21]. P50 auditory sensory gating is elicited by presenting a pair of acoustic stimuli separated by short inter-stimulus intervals. The first stimulus of the pair elicits the initial P50 neural activity, and the second stimulus of the pair measures the filtering or the gating process [24]. This filtering processing is reflected by the amount of neural inhibition where the P50 amplitude will be reduced from the stimulation of the second acoustic stimulus of the pair. Auditory sensory gating from P50 is measured by the differences in the P50 amplitudes elicited from the first stimulus of the pair and the second stimulus of the pair. It is thought that the P50 from the second stimulus of the pair triggered the neural inhibition because of the short inter-stimulus interval from the first stimulus of the pair. This short inter-stimulus interval is shorter than the neural recovery period thus causing a reduction in the P50 amplitude. The lack of auditory sensory gating differences between the first stimulus and second stimulus of the pair is associated with auditory sensory gating deficit. Auditory sensory gating deficit from P50 assessment was found in patients with attention deficit hyperactivity disorder (ADHD) [10], schizophrenia [13], and an autism spectrum disorder [11]. Early identification of auditory sensory gating deficit in children can serve as a predictive measure of future mental health issues as shown in the previous literature [25].

3.2 Electrophysiology test: ABR sensory gating

Few studies in the last 10 years have reported the potential to measure auditory sensory gating from the auditory efferent pathways by eliciting auditory brainstem response (ABR) and modulating the ABRs using attentional tasks [19, 22, 23]. These findings were inconsistent with some of the earlier studies that found no significant influence of the attention to the ABR findings thus dismissing the neural inhibition activities that occur in the efferent pathway between the level of the auditory cortex and the brainstem [26, 27].

To record an ABR with attention modulation, the participant needs to perform certain psychological tasks while the ABR is being acquired. Among psychological tasks that have been used in the ABR acquisition are the working memory task [23], Stroop task [19, 22] (see Section 3), and visual and auditory discrimination tasks [26]. Stroop task has been used to measure auditory sensory gating in recent studies [19, 22]. In this auditory sensory gating test, the patients are required to count the frequency of congruent and incongruent digits while the ABR is acquired from the patient. For congruent, the digit is consistent with the frequency of the digit presented, for example, number 3 is presented 3 times (*333*). For incongruent, the digit is not consistent with the frequency of digit presented, such as digit of 3 are presented 5 times (*33333*). The ABR wave V amplitude will reduce when the study participants are introduced with cognitive interference elements like the incongruent numbers; this is related to the auditory sensory gating inhibition.

Two recent studies investigated the influence of cognitive interference using ABR concurrent with Stroop task in adults. In the first study, Brännström et al. [19] recorded the ABR waveforms using 3000 Hz tone burst stimulus in twenty adult subjects together with active Stroop task procedure. The authors found the ABR wave V amplitudes did not change with the presence of cognitive interference in comparison with the baseline ABR. However, the authors identified a significant relationship between the response time and the ABR wave V amplitude. In detail, as the response time increases by the cognitive interference, it follows with a reduction in the ABR wave V amplitude, suggesting that cognitive interference is in proportion with the neural inhibition. In addition, Brännström et al. [19] also found some of their subjects showed significantly larger inhibition and some did not, which suggests auditory sensory gating abilities are varied between subjects. Dzulkarnain et al. [22] studied the influence of cognitive interference on the ABR findings in 23 adult participants that were further categorized as Huffaz and non-Huffaz. Similar to Brännström et al. [19] findings, the authors found no significant difference in the ABR wave V amplitude with and without cognitive interference in both within and between groups analysis. The authors also found only half of their study participants had a significant neural inhibition from the high cognitive interference activities.

4. New findings

To date, studies that investigated the influence of cognitive interference or auditory sensory gating using ABR are only limited to the adult as the study participants. To the author's knowledge, there is no known study that investigates the influence of cognitive interference in the children population. The ABR results with cognitive interference from the adult population may not be applicable to the children population possibly due to the differences in their structure and function of the auditory system, particularly at the auditory cortex and circuits surrounding them, and it may take up to the age of 20 years to reach full maturation state [28]. Because of that, a study to understand the auditory sensory gating mechanism in the children population is required.

In this chapter, preliminary data obtained from ten typically developing children (age between 8 and 12 years old) is presented. This study aims to investigate the auditory sensory gating mechanism using ABR with cognitive interference specifically using Stroop interference task in children. A case study on ABR sensory gating was later described. The case study was conducted in a mild autism spectrum disorder child and a comparison with a typically developing child was made.

All children had normal hearing and middle ear function based on their pure tone audiometry and tympanometry findings. The study took place in the electrophysiology room of the International Islamic University Malaysia (IIUM) Hearing and Speech Clinic. ABRs were acquired from the study participants at 70 dBnHL using 1000 Hz alternating tone-burst stimulus with 2-0-2 stimulus envelope and Blackman gating function (4 milliseconds duration). Ipsilateral electrode montage was used to record the ABR neural activities at 20 milliseconds time window with stimulus repetition rate set at 33.1 Hz. No contralateral masking noise was applied since minimal cross-over was anticipated when using 3A insert earphone. The recording was conducted using the Interacoustic Eclipse auditory evoked potential system. The ABR signals were averaged using the Bayesian averaging technique until the Stroop task procedure completed with a minimum of 2000 sweeps. The ABR was filtered using a 3000–30 Hz bandpass filter and any signals that exceeded 40 μV were rejected by the automatic artifact rejection system.

During the ABR acquisition, the participant performed Stroop counting-digit task procedure as outlined in Section 3. **Table 1** summarized the test items used in each Stroop task condition (congruent, incongruent, and neutral). These test items were randomly presented and were set to only 52 trials for each Stroop task condition that later corresponds to the final number of ABR sweeps at the end of the recording. In short, the total number of ABR sweeps was determined by the duration for each participant to complete each of the Stroop task test condition (congruent, incongruent, and neutral). Stroop counting-digit task was created using E-Prime version 3.0 software and the digit was displayed on the screen of a laptop. As highlighted in Section 3, participants need to count the frequency of the digit or character while ignoring the actual number itself. Subsequently, they need to press the frequency of the digit in the number series using the appropriate "key" on the keyboard of a laptop.

4.1 Preliminary findings

4.1.1 Data analysis

The analysis of this study focuses on the ABR wave V peak, specifically its absolute latencies, amplitudes, and the amount of neural inhibition. The ABR absolute latencies are determined from the onset of the stimulus until the time it took for the action potential to produce the peak of ABR wave V. The amplitude of wave V was determined from the peak of wave V to the preceding trough. The amount of neural inhibition or ABR sensory gating was determined from the amplitude of ABR wave V from the incongruent condition minus the amplitude of ABR wave V from the neutral

	Stroop task conditions		
	Congruent	**Incongruent**	**Neutral**
Test items	• 1 • 22 • 333 • 4444	• 11 • 111 • 1111 • 2 • 222 • 2222 • 3 • 33 • 3333 • 4 • 44 • 444	• # • ## • ### • ####

Table 1.
The test items used in each Stroop task condition (congruent, incongruent, and neutral).

test condition. The percentage of the neural inhibition was calculated from the formula recommended by Dzulkarnain et al. [22]. The percentage of correct responses that indicates the percentage of trials that were correctly identified in each Stroop task condition was also calculated. The reaction time that indicates the time taken by the child to provide the answer was also analyzed. Stroop interference for both reaction time and percentage of correct response was also computed from the differences in the Stroop task results of incongruent and neutral test conditions.

There was no significant difference ($p > 0.05$) in the ABR wave V amplitudes and latencies between the ABRs recorded under incongruent test condition (latencies: M = 7.46, SD = 0.57; amplitudes: M = 0.63, SD = 0.18) and neutral test condition (latencies: M = 7.54, SD = 0.90; amplitudes: M = 0.70, SD = 0.24) consistent with small effect size ($d < 0.3$). In general, this result indicates there was no significant influence of the cognitive interference on the ABR wave V amplitudes and latencies. The result also showed no significant difference ($p > 0.05$) in the percentage of correct response and reaction time between incongruent test condition and neutral test condition with moderate effect size ($d < 0.5$) as shown in **Table 2**.

No significant relationship was identified for Stroop interference for reaction time and percentage of the correct response with the ABR sensory gating ($p > 0.05$). **Table 3** shows the percentage of wave V reduction following with cognitive interference in each study participant. Of the 10 study participants, 8 children show a reduction in their ABR wave V amplitude from the incongruent cognitive load and interference task. Although neural inhibition can be seen in the majority of the study participants, statistically, cognitive interference has no influence on the ABR findings in children as shown in this study.

4.1.2 Case study

Figure 1 shows the ABR waveforms recorded from 1 typically developing child (age: 6-year-old) and autism spectrum disorder (ASD) child (age: 9-year-old) under three Stroop task conditions.

	Incongruent	Neutral	P-value	Effect size
% correct response	99.02% (1.67)	99.41% (1.32)	0.17	0.26
Reaction time (milliseconds)	1038.25 (193.73)	964.39 (145.97)	0.19	0.43

Table 2.
Percentage of correct response and reaction time in Stroop incongruent and neutral conditions.

Subject ID	Incongruent minus neutral ABR wave V amplitude (μV)%
101	1.7
102	−40.09
103	68.05
104	−10.97
105	−14.32
106	29.98
107	−12.12
108	−20.66
109	−27.81
110	−7.18

Table 3.
Percentage of ABR wave V amplitude reduction Following cognitive interference in all subjects.

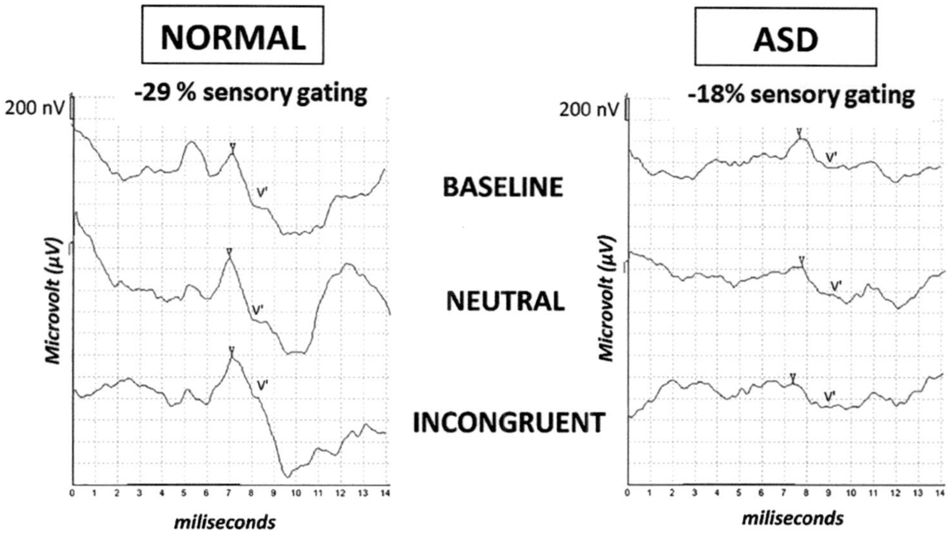

Figure 1.
The ABR waveforms recorded from 1 typically developing child (age: 6-year-old) and autism spectrum disorder (ASD) child (age: 9-year-old) under three Stroop task conditions.

Table 4 shows the Stroop-counting digit results in both ASD children and typical developing children. Results showed that the ASD child (-18%) has less inhibition or lower ABR sensory gating amplitude than a typically normal developing child (-29%) when comparisons of the ABR amplitude between those under

	ASD	TD
Reaction time (milliseconds)	1173	782
Correct response (%)	98%	100%
Stroop interference reaction time (milliseconds)	413	129
Stroop interference correct response (%)	−1.67	0

ASD: Autism spectrum disorder; TD, typical developing child.

Table 4.
The Stroop counting digit results in autism and typically developing child.

cognitive interference (incongruent) and without cognitive interference (neutral) was made descriptively. The ASD child also had a longer reaction time and a lower percentage of correct Stroop task responses under the Stroop task with cognitive interference (incongruent) than the typically normal developing child. In addition, the ASD child had also lower Stroop interference effects for the percentage of correct response but higher Stroop interference effect for reaction time descriptively. Overall, this case study showed that ASD children took a longer time to do the Stroop task under cognitive interference test conditions and this corresponds with a lower neural inhibition as shown by their ABR findings. This case study indicates a promising finding for future research if more data are collected for both normal and ASD children.

5. Summary and future direction

Our preliminary data in children have shown that the auditory brainstem response was not affected by the cognitive interference in typically developing children. Having said that, the majority of the study participants' ABRs showed evidence of neural inhibition, following cognitive interference. In general, our preliminary data partly coincide with Brännström et al. [19] findings that found an association between cognitive interference with the reduction in the ABR amplitude.

While our findings were inconclusive to relate the cognitive inhibition from the auditory cortex efferent pathways with the reduction in the neural activity at the brainstem, a few considerations should be taken in the future study to better understand the auditory sensory gating mechanism. One of the considerations is to ensure the residual noise level is kept constant throughout the ABRs recording among the Stroop task conditions. It is a well-known fact that the ABR amplitude is highly influenced by noise and therefore the conclusion of the study can be confounded by this factor. Next, future studies need to consider the ABR test-retest reliability values as an indicator of whether truly clinical changes have occurred in the ABR findings [29]. The third consideration is to explore the ABR recorded with cognitive interference among patients with known sensory gating deficit such as ADHD, autism, or schizophrenia since our case study has given some indication that differences may exist in the ABR sensory gating findings between a typically developing child and those with potential sensory gating deficits.

Acknowledgements

This work was supported by the Transdisciplinary Research Grant Scheme (TRGS/1/2019/UIAM/02/4/2) from the Ministry of Higher Education of Malaysia.

The work of this study had been presented at the 2021 International Evoked Response Audiometry IERASG conference.

Conflict of interest

The authors declare no conflict of interests.

Author details

Ahmad Aidil Arafat Dzulkarnain[1*], Nur Hafizah Sulaiman[1], Fatin Amira Shahrudin[1], Shahrul Na'im Sidek[2], Hazlina Md. Yusof[2] and Madihah Khalid[3]

1 Department of Audiology and Speech-Language Pathology, Kulliyyah of Allied Health Sciences, International Islamic University Malaysia, Kuantan, Pahang, Malaysia

2 Department of Mechatronic Engineering, Kulliyyah of Engineering, International Islamic University Malaysia, Kuala Lumpur, Malaysia

3 Department of Curriculum and Instruction, Kulliyyah of Education, Kulliyyah of Education, International Islamic University Malaysia, Kuala Lumpur, Malaysia

*Address all correspondence to: a.aidil@gmail.com

References

[1] Liu X, Zhang O, Chen A, Hu K, Ehret G, Yan J. Corticofugal augmentation of the auditory brainstem response with respect to cortical preference. Frontiers in Systems Neuroscience. 2019;**13**:39

[2] Schofield BR, Beebe NL. Descending auditory pathways and plasticity. In: The Oxford Handbook of the Auditory Brainstem. Oxford, England: Oxford University Press; 2019

[3] Hood, LJ. Clinical Applications of the Auditory Brainstem Response, San Diego, London: Singular Publishing; 1998

[4] Moller AR, Jannetta PJ, Moller MB. Neural generators of brainstem evoked potentials. Results from human intracranial recordings. Annals of Otology, Rhinology and Laryngology. 1981;**90**(6 Pt 1):591-596

[5] Malmierca E, Nuñez A. Corticofugal action on somatosensory response properties of rat nucleus gracilis cells. Brain Research. 1998;**810**(1-2):172-180

[6] Nuñez A, Malmierca E. Corticofugal Modulation of Sensory Information. Berlin, Heidelberg: Springer; 2007

[7] Hetrick WP, Erickson MA, Smith DA. Phenomenological dimensions of sensory gating. Schizophrenia Bulletin. 2012;**38**(1):178-191

[8] McGhie A, Chapman J. Disorders of attention and perception in early schizophrenia. British Journal of Medical Psychology. 1961;**34**(2):103-116

[9] Jones L, Hills PJ, Dick KM, Jones SP, Bright P. Cognitive mechanisms associated with auditory sensory gating. Brain and Cognition. 2016;**102**:33-45

[10] Durukan I et al. P50 sensory gating in children and adolescents with ADHD and effects of methylphenidate administration on P50 sensory gating. Bulletin of Clinical Psychopharmacology. 2011;**21**(1):42-48

[11] Orekhova EV, Stroganova TA, Prokofyev AO, Nygren G, Gillberg C, Elam M. Sensory gating in young children with autism: Relation to age, IQ, and EEG gamma oscillations. Neuroscience Letters. 2008;**434**(2):218-223

[12] Mei Lv M et al. Study on p50 sensory gating in children with autism spectrum disorders in Shanghai. North American Journal of Medicine and Science. 2014;7(3):103-106

[13] Sánchez-Morla EM, Santos JL, Aparicio A, García-Jiménez MÁ, Soria C, Arango C. Neuropsychological correlates of P50 sensory gating in patients with schizophrenia. Schizophrenia Research. 2013;**143**(1):102-106

[14] Bunney WE Jr et al. Structured interview for assessing perceptual anomalies (SIAPA). Schizophrenia Bulletin. 1999;**25**(3):577-592

[15] Jusoh M. The effects of sound-cognitive training intervention to the sensory gating abilities and working memory skill in children with attention deficit hyperactivity disorders symptoms [Doctor of Philosophy (PhD) thesis]. Pahang, Malaysia: Department of Audiology and Speech-Language Pathology, International Islamic University Malaysia; 2020

[16] Green EJ, Barber PJ. Interference effects in an auditory Stroop task: Congruence and correspondence. Acta Psychologica. 1983;**53**(3):183-194

[17] Stroop JR. Studies of interference in serial verbal reactions. Journal of Experimental Psychology. 1935;**18**(6):643

[18] Bush G, Whalen PJ, Shin LM, Rauch SL. The counting Stroop: A cognitive interference task. Nature Protocols. 2006;**1**(1):230-233

[19] Brännström KJ, Wilson WJ, Waechter S. Increasing cognitive interference modulates the amplitude of the auditory brainstem response. Journal of the American Academy of Audiology. 2018;**29**(06):512-519

[20] Hall J III. eHandbook of Auditory Evoked Responses: Principles, Procedures & Protocols. Pretoria: Pearson; 2015

[21] Baker N et al. Neurophysiological assessment of sensory gating in psychiatric inpatients: Comparison between schizophrenia and other diagnoses. Biological Psychiatry. 1987;**22**(5):603-617

[22] Dzulkarnain AA, Azizi AK, Sulaiman NH. Auditory sensory gating in Huffaz using an auditory brainstem response with a psychological task: A preliminary investigation. Journal of Taibah University Medical Sciences. 2020;**15**(6):495-501

[23] Sörqvist P, Stenfelt S, Rönnberg J. Working memory capacity and visual–verbal cognitive load modulate auditory–sensory gating in the brainstem: Toward a unified view of attention. Journal of Cognitive Neuroscience. 2012;**24**(11):2147-2154

[24] Siegel C, Waldo M, Mizner G, Adler LE, Freedman R. Deficits in sensory gating in schizophrenic patients and their relatives: Evidence obtained with auditory evoked responses. Archives of General Psychiatry. 1984;**41**(6):607-612

[25] Hutchison AK, Hunter SK, Wagner BD, Calvin EA, Zerbe GO, Ross RG. Diminished infant P50 sensory gating predicts increased 40-month-old attention, anxiety/depression, and externalizing symptoms. Journal of Attention Disorders. 2017;**21**(3):209-218

[26] Kuk FK, Abbas PJ. Effects of attention on the auditory evoked potentials recorded from the vertex (ABR) and the promontory (CAP) of human listeners. Neuropsychologia. 1989;**27**(5):665-673

[27] Lukas JH. The role of efferent inhibition in human auditory attention: An examination of the auditory brainstem potentials. International Journal of Neuroscience. 1981;**12**(2):137-145

[28] Ponton CW, Eggermont JJ, Kwong B, Don M. Maturation of human central auditory system activity: Evidence from multi-channel evoked potentials. Clinical Neurophysiology. 2000;**111**(2):220-236

[29] Jamal FN, Dzulkarnain AAA, Shahrudin FA, Marzuki MN. Test-retest reliability of level-specific CE-chirp auditory brainstem response in normal-hearing adults. Journal of Audiology & Otology. 2021;**25**(1):14

Section 3

Auditory Disorders and Involved Genes

Chapter 6

A Short Overview on Hearing Loss and Related Auditory Defects

Hina Khan, Hafiza Idrees, Zunaira Munir and Memoona Ramzan

Abstract

Hearing is the ability of a person to recognize sound in the surroundings and it makes communication possible. Ear is the human organ serving as a transducer that perceives signals from the environment and converts it into detectable forms for interpretation by the brain. The auditory system is among one of the most highly studied systems. Researchers have described the physiological function of the system in detail but due to its complexity, the genetic mechanisms and genes implicated in auditory function are still being revealed. Numerous studies on the genetics of hearing indicate hearing loss as one of the most common and prevalent disorders as it affects approximately five million people worldwide. Besides hearing loss, there are several other pathologies of auditory system which are common and have an established genetic basis. In this chapter, we will introduce the genetics of some common auditory pathologies including syndromic and non-syndromic hearing loss, auditory neuropathy, age-related hearing loss, and tinnitus. These understandings will 1 day lead to better diagnosis, management, and cures.

Keywords: auditory neuropathy, hearing loss, tinnitus

1. Introduction

The medical condition which affects any process during sound transmission from ear to brain i.e. anywhere along the auditory pathway is termed hearing loss or deafness [1, 2]. The range of normal audible spectrum is 20–20,000 Hz. Hearing loss is the third most prevalent physical condition and one of the most common sensory disorders in humans [3, 4]. According to World Health Organization (WHO) (http://www.who.int/), around 466 million people (or 6.1% of the world's population) are affected by deafness, including 34 million children under the age of 15 and 50% of all adults over the age of 75 [5]. By 2030, this figure is expected to increase to 630 million, and by 2050, it will be over 900 million [6].

Defective hearing can be categorized into a variety of types based on the damaged area of the auditory system, severity, type, age, mode of inheritance, and/or the involvement of other phenotypes. By severity, the hearing loss may be mild (20–40 dB HL), moderate (41–70 dB HL), severe (71–95 dB HL), and profound deafness that is greater than 95 dB HL [7]. Hearing loss can be classified on the basis of involved regions of the ear as well. Conductive hearing loss describes the phenotype due to the outer or middle ear defects. Sensorineural hearing loss involves inner ear defects. Mixed hearing loss indicates the presence of conductive and sensorineural hearing loss together [8]. With reference to age, hearing loss may be pre-lingual in which hearing loss occurs before speech development, or post-lingual in which hearing loss occurs after speech development [9].

Hearing loss can be genetic or caused by environmental factors. Environmental factors include high exposure to ototoxic agents, trauma, and bacterial or viral infections [10]. Genetic hearing loss can be inherited in different modes. It can include autosomal dominant, autosomal recessive, X-linked, or mitochondrial modes of inheritance. Mitochondrial hearing loss accounts for less than 1% of all instances of hereditary hearing loss. A human mitochondrion's genome is 16,569-bp long and contains 22 tRNA and 2 rRNA genes and encodes 13 proteins. Mitochondrial hearing loss may be non-syndromic or syndromic as some other associated disorders can occur in addition to hearing [11]. X-linked hearing loss accounts for around 1–2% of cases of non-syndromic hearing loss, as well as many syndromic types. Approximately 80% of inherited hearing loss is autosomal recessive. Predominantly, it is a monogenic trait in each family. However, overall, it is heterogenetic [12]. Genetic hearing loss can be either in the form of syndromic or non-syndromic form. Approximately 30% of deafness comprises syndromic forms. It involves the presence of hearing loss in combination with other symptoms. More than 400 syndromes are known to be associated with deafness as one of the phenotypes and many of the causative genes involved in these syndromes have been identified [13]. Most common syndromes which are associated with hearing loss are Pendred syndrome and Usher syndrome [14].

Predominantly, 70% of deafness is non-syndromic i.e. hearing loss is the only phenotype. Approximately, 80% of all non-syndromic deafness cases are autosomal recessive (DFNB), 15–20% are autosomal dominant (DFNA), 1–2% cases are X-linked (DFN) and less than 1% of hearing loss is Y linked (DFNY) or mitochondrial [15]. More than 115 non-syndromic hearing loss genes have been identified (https://hereditaryhearingloss.org, accessed April 2022). More than 100 loci have been mapped to different chromosomal positions for non-syndromic autosomal recessive hearing loss in humans. It was originally estimated that approximately 1% of human protein-coding genes are involved in audition [16], but this number has already been exceeded. New research indicates that up to a thousand genes may be involved in hearing. Therefore, additional genes remain to be discovered that cause hearing loss.

2. Syndromic hearing loss

Syndromic hearing loss is defined as hearing loss accompanying other clinical features in at least one other body system [17]. Up to 30% of hereditary deafness is syndromic and more than 400 genetic disorders have been associated with hearing loss [18]. There are many syndromes associated with hearing loss, but the most common hearing loss-linked syndromes are Pendred syndrome, Usher syndrome, and Waardenburg syndrome [19]. Pendred and Usher syndrome are often confused with non-syndromic cases due to delayed onset of subtle manifestation of other phenotypes.

Pendred syndrome is a condition typically associated with sensorineural deafness, goiter (an enlargement of the thyroid gland), and/or enlarged vestibular aqueduct. It is the most common autosomal recessive sensorineural hearing loss with an estimated incidence of 10 in 100,000 individuals [20–22]. The hearing impairment is usually congenital or has early-onset while goiter appears in the later years of life. Pendred syndrome is mainly caused by the biallelic variants in *SLC26A4* gene, which encodes Pendrin, a transmembrane exchanger of anions and bases. Until now, numerous missense, deletions, and truncating variants in *SLC26A4* for Pendred syndrome have been reported [23]. Splice-site, as well as a few missense variants, are described in association with non-syndromic hearing impairment, DFNB4 [24]. Additionally, there are some variants, which may cause non-syndromic deafness DFNB4 or syndromic PDS in a few cases [25].

Usher syndrome is a condition characterized by deafness/hearing loss and vision/an eye disease called retinitis pigmentosa (RP); sometimes also affecting balance. It is the second most syndrome associated with hearing loss with a frequency of 6 in 100,000 individuals, and is often misdiagnosed and presented as a non-syndromic disorder [26]. Usher syndrome has three main clinical types based on the age of onset and audiovestibular features. Usher syndrome presents significant genetic heterogeneity, which means more than one gene can cause the same type of the syndrome [17]. Usher type I (USH1) is the most severe subtype, characterized by profound congenital sensorineural deafness, progressive retinitis pigmentosa, and vestibular dysfunction. To date, five USH1 genes have been identified; *MYO7A* (the most common), *CDH23* (second most common), *PCDH15* (third most common), USH1C, and USH1G (minor effects) which are implicated at the loci *USH1B*, *USH1D*, *USH1F*, *USH1C*, and *USH1G* respectively [27].

Usher type II (USH2) is characterized by moderate to severe hearing loss, later onset of retinal pigmentosa and normal vestibular function. Three genetic loci have been involved in USH2, namely, *USH2A*, *USH2C,* and *USH2D* along with the corresponding genes. In Usher type III (USH3), hearing loss is progressive, postlingual, and retinal pigmentosa and the vestibular dysfunction are more variable [26]. Some atypical genes and loci have been related to the disease; however, their roles are not very well studied, for example, *ESPN* (USH1M), *HARS* (USH3), *CEP78* (atypical Usher), *CEP250* (atypical Usher), *ABDH12* (USH3), and *ARSG* (atypical Usher, USH4), and three loci, namely, *USH1E*, *USH1H*, and *USH1K* [28]. As the Usher type II and III are usually associated with moderate to severe hearing loss and retinitis pigmentosa developed in later stages of life, these two types of Usher syndrome are often misdiagnosed as non-syndromic moderate to severe hearing loss [29].

Waardenburg syndrome (WS) is also known as an auditory-pigmentary disorder as it is characterized by hearing loss along with pigmentation abnormalities in skin, hair, and eyes. WS is the most common type of autosomal dominant sensorineural hearing loss with an occurrence of 1 in 40,000 individuals. Based on clinical features, WS has 4 subtypes; Type I, II, III, and IV and six genes *PAX3*, *MITF*, *SNAI2*, *EDN3*, *EDNRB*, and *SOX10* have been identified. Type II patients present typical hearing loss and pigment abnormalities while types I, III, and IV are associated with some additional symptoms affecting face, limb, and/or gastrointestinal system [30, 31].

Variants of many genes are involved in both syndromic and non-syndromic hearing loss. The phenotypic variability caused by the same variant can be due to the influence of genetic or environmental modifiers. Some of the syndromic deafness phenotypes are age-dependent and cannot be diagnosed in children; for example, retinitis pigmentosa development in Usher syndrome. The list of syndromes associated with hearing loss is large but here we have listed only the most common ones [32].

3. Non-syndromic hearing loss

Non-syndromic hearing loss, deafness without any other defects, is highly heterogeneous [33]. Genetic studies and linkage analysis have been helpful in identifying genes involved in hearing loss. Reports till 2021 indicate a total of 124 genes that have been identified for non-syndromic hearing loss. Among these, 78 genes are involved in autosomal recessive non-syndromic hearing loss while 51 genes cause autosomal dominant non-syndromic hearing loss (**Figure 1**). About 5 genes are known to cause non-syndromic deafness in an X-linked manner [34] (https://hereditaryhearingloss.org/, accessed April 2022).

3.1 Autosomal recessive non-syndromic hearing loss (ARNSHL)

Worldwide data, with the prominence of Caucasian populations, indicate that *GJB2* variants account for the maximal cases of autosomal recessive non-syndromic deafness with the rate exceeding 50% of reported cases. *SLC26A4* is the second in line causative gene followed by *MYO15A*, *OTOF*, *CDH23*, and *TMC1* [35].

In this section, we will shed light on the most common genes involved in autosomal recessive non-syndromic hearing loss (ARNSHL).

DFNB1 is the first deafness locus that was mapped in 1994 [36]. *GJB2* encoding connexin26 (Cx26) was assigned to this locus during the study on three autosomal recessive non-syndromic sensorineural deaf families with nonsense variants in the gene. Connexin26 plays an important role in human ear development. The immunohistochemical staining of human cochlear cells has revealed high levels of *GJB2* expression [37]. Cx26 being a gap junction protein regulates intracellular communication and plays an important role in maintaining potassium levels in the inner ear. This potassium balance is crucial to normal auditory function [38]. Over the years, several studies have been conducted for the development of efficient therapy targeting hereditary hearing loss. A study showed that introducing normal *GJB2* gene through bacterial artificial chromosome (BAC) in *GJB2* deleted mice resulted in normal hearing and Auditory Brain Response (ABR) score [39]. Variants in *GJB2* cause approximately 16% of deafness in Iran [40]. In Pakistan, *GJB2*-related deafness frequency ranges from 6

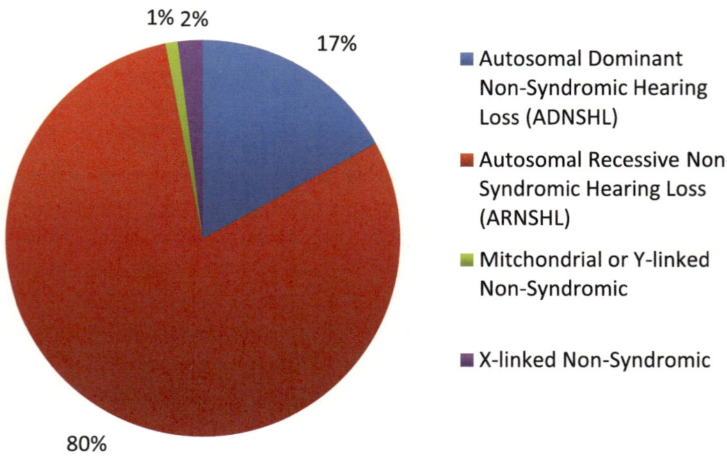

Figure 1.
Frequency of various inheritance patterns for non-syndromic hearing loss.

to 7% for profound deafness [41] to 9.5% for moderate to severe hearing loss [42]. The variant c.35delG is the most common bi-allelic *GJB2* mutation worldwide with allele frequency up to 100% in European, North African, and Middle Eastern populations [43]. However, different variants are more common in other populations.

DFNB4 is caused by variants in *SLC26A4*, causing both autosomal recessive Pendred syndrome as well as non-syndromic deafness. It was first identified as a Pendred syndrome gene (PDS) using a positional cloning strategy. A year later, the gene was found to cause non-syndromic autosomal recessive deafness when a consanguineous family in southwest India was studied having a variant in the Pendred gene with no symptoms of goiter [44, 45]. Up till now 641 variants in *SLC26A4* have been reported in public databases (http://www.hgmd.cf.ac.uk/ac/search.php). *SLC26A4* encodes pendrin, an exchange of bicarbonate/chloride ions in the inner ear maintaining the homeostasis of endolymph [46]. The role of pendrin in normal hearing is elucidated by the fact that knockout mice *Slc26a4*$^{-/-}$ are completely deaf with vestibular dysfunction [47]. In knockout mice, reduced pH and utricular endolymphatic potential along with an increased level of Ca^{2+} are key factors leading to deafness. As it seems obvious, low Ca^{2+} concentration in human ear endolymph is crucial to the normal hearing process [48]. In a cohort of patients, single allele variants in *SLC26A4* fail to account for DFNB4 or Pendred syndrome. Digenic variants for some genes along with *SLC26A4* have been reported to be causative in such cases. *KCNJ10* an inwardly rectifying K^+ channel gene is important for maintaining endocochlear potential. Heterozygous variants in both *SLC26A4* and *KCNJ10* result in digenic non-syndromic hearing loss associated with enlarged vestibular aqueduct syndrome [49]. Similarly, missense *EPHA2* variant in patients with mono-allelic *SLC26A4* variations has been reported in patients with Pendred syndrome. EPHA2 controls pendrin localization by forming a complex with it and faulty EPHA2 causes mislocalization of pendrin in the inner ear [50].

DFNB3, a non-syndromic deafness locus maps to chromosome 17p11.2. *MYO15A* pertaining to this locus causes congenital profound deafness in humans and *shaker2* (*sh2*) phenotype with vestibular defects in mice [51–53]. MYO15A encoded by this gene is an unconventional Myosin; tail homology 4—protein 4.1, ezrin, radixin, and moesin (MyTH4-FERM) myosin [54]. MYO15A is localized at the tips of both the outer hair cells (OHCs) and the inner hair cells (IHCs) and has a developmental role in the formation of stereocilia and thus, is indispensable to the hearing process [55]. Although, identified as a gene for profound deafness, less severe cases of hearing loss due to *MYO15A* variants are well known. The severity of deafness due to variants in this gene is in accordance with the protein domain being affected [56]. Frequency of *MYO15A*-related deafness is 5.71% in the Iranian population [57] and about 7.2% in the Vietnamese population [58].

Deafness autosomal recessive non-syndromic deafness, DFNB9 is caused by *OTOF* gene encoding otoferlin protein [59]. Otoferlin is essential to human hearing as it plays a role in inner hair cell formation and exocytosis of synaptic vesicles at the auditory inner hair cell ribbon synapse [60]. Otoferlin converts low-intensity stimuli at the synapse between inner hair cells and auditory nerve fiber [61]. *OTOF* variants cause auditory neuropathy (discussed later in this chapter) manifested as severe to profound non-syndromic deafness in most individuals. Cochlear implants in patients with *OTOF*-related deafness have shown promising results [62, 63].

CDH23 was identified in families with Usher syndrome (USH1D) mapping to *DFNB12* locus [64]. Immuno-histochemical studies on rodent models showed localization of cadherin to upper and lower tip-links. These tip-links lie near stereocilia of hair cells and gate mechanoelectrical transduction [65]. The phenotype due to mutations in *CDH23* depends upon the type of variants in the gene. Missense variants with residual protein function are thought to cause DFNB12 while homozygous nonsense, frameshift, splice site, and a few missense variants with total loss of function cause *USH1D* [66]. Cochlear implants in children aged 11–36 months with *CDH23* mutations improved their hearing, speech, and performance necessitating the need for early diagnosis and possible improvement in hearing following implants [67].

TMC1 variants are responsible for both dominant form of deafness DFNA36 as well as non-syndromic recessive hearing loss DFNB7/B11 [68]. Most of the *TMC1* variants cause autosomal recessive non-syndromic deafness while only a few are involved in dominantly inherited hearing loss. TMC1 is a transmembrane channel protein that forms the pore of mechanosensory transduction channels (MET) in vertebrate inner ear hair cells [69]. In Pakistani population, 3.4% of autosomal recessive non-syndromic hearing loss (ARSNHL) is caused by *TMC1* variants [70]. The *TMC1*-related ARSNHL is 3.1% of diagnosed cases in the western European population [71] while 4.3–8.1% in the Turkish population [72, 73].

In countries like Pakistan where consanguinity rate is high, gene variants of *HGF*, *MYO7A*, *TMPRSS3*, *CIB2*, and *CLDN14* along with the ones mentioned above also contribute to large cases of profound and moderate to severe hearing loss [74, 75]. *HGF* within *DFNB39* locus 7q21.11 encodes hepatocyte growth factor. The variants of *HGF*, responsible for autosomal-recessive, non-syndromic hearing loss are located in intron 4. Also, indels in a highly conserved 3′ untranslated region (3′UTR) affect splicing of *HGF* exons resulting in deafness [76].

MYO7A mapping to 11q13.5 causes non-syndromic hearing loss both in recessive and dominant fashion and Usher syndrome (USH1B). MYO7A the unconventional myosin is required for the normal function of cochlear hair cells [77, 78].

TMPRSS3 variants cause pre-lingual hearing impairment i.e. DFNB10 and late-onset DFNB8-associated hearing impairment. The severity of phenotype depends upon the combination of two mutant alleles. The type II transmembrane protease 3 encoded by *TMPRSS3* regulates epithelial sodium channels and potassium calcium-activated channel subfamily M alpha 1 (KCNMA1). Enac (Epithelial Amiloride Sensitive Sodium Channel) in turn controls the signaling pathway in inner ear essential to hearing. In the human ear, *TMPRSS3* variants lead to hair cell apoptosis and disruption of intracellular homeostasis [79–83].

3.2 Autosomal dominant non-syndromic hearing loss

In the case of autosomal dominant non-syndromic hearing loss, frequently reported genes in literature include *WFS1*, *KCNQ4*, *COCH*, and *GJB2* although dominant hearing loss does not account for a large number of cases as compared to autosomal recessive deafness [35].

DFNA2 (Deafness autosomal dominant 2A) locus was assigned to cause autosomal dominant non-syndromic hearing loss (ADNSHL) by Kubisch et al. [84]. *KCNQ4* mapping to this locus encodes Potassium Voltage-Gated Channel Subfamily Q Member 4 protein expressed in OHCs in cochlea. Variants of *KCNQ4* implicated in ADNSHL disrupt the channel's ability to differentiate between K^+ and Na^+ ions and exert a strong dominant-negative effect on K+ currents in the inner ear [84].

Interestingly, *KCNQ4* variant has also been reported to cause hearing loss in a pseudo-dominant fashion. In a family with genetic heterogeneity, pathogenic variant c.872C > T in a homozygous state caused early-onset moderate to profound or moderate to severe deafness that progressed to profound deafness in a patient. This variant in heterozygous state caused mild to moderate hearing loss in the carrier [85]. In another study, *KCNQ4* gene variant c.1044_1051del8 was identified to be responsible for causing autosomal recessive hearing loss with a severe phenotype [86]. *KCNQ4* variants c.211delC, c.725G > A, and c.1044_1051del8 induce cell death in heterologous expression systems in a dominant manner [87]. Recent studies propose possible contribution of *KCNQ4* to age-related deafness as well [88].

COCH mapping to 14q12 was described to cause DFNA9 with vestibular dysfunction in three unrelated families [89]. In DFNA9, pathogenic variants of *COCH* lead to the accumulation of acellular deposits in the inner ear due to gain of function of mutant cochlin. Cochlin protein is the major component of interossicular joints and tympanic membrane of middle ear [90]. For many years, it was thought to be a gene implicated only for autosomal dominant hearing loss, when in 2018 a homozygous nonsense variant in *COCH* was identified to cause congenital prelingual recessive deafness DFNB110 [91].

WSF1 was identified as a gene for Wolfram syndrome; an autosomal recessive disorder, by a positional cloning approach [92]. In 2001, Bespalova et al. defined families associated with autosomal dominant non-syndromic low-frequency sensorineural hearing loss (NSLFHL), DFNA6/14/38 having variants in *WSF1* gene [93].

GJB2 has already been described for autosomal recessive non-syndromic hearing loss. The dominant mode of inheritance for *GJB2* was proposed in deaf families with palmoplantar keratoderma [37, 94]. The role of *GJB2* for autosomal dominant deafness 3A (DFNA3) was defined in a study on *GJB2* variants in the Austrian population [95].

3.3 X-linked non-syndromic hearing loss

The prevalence of X-linked non-syndromic deafness is 1–3%. As males are hemizygous for X-chromosome, they are predominantly affected by X-linked deafness [11].

Loss of function variants in *PRPS1* encoding phosphoribosyl pyrophosphate (PRPP) synthetase 1 enzyme was assigned to non-syndromic X-linked sensorineural deafness, DFNX1, in a Chinese family [96]. Another gene for X-linked non-syndromic deafness, *POU3F4* was defined by De kok et al. Nonsense mutations in *SMPX*, c.109G > T in a German family and c.175G > T in a Spanish family were assigned to *DFNX4* locus for X-linked non-syndromic deafness [97]. *AIFM1* pathogenic variants are involved in familial and sporadic cases of X-linked recessive auditory neuropathy spectrum disorder [98]. Single mutations in *COL4A6* were linked to a genetic disorder when a pathogenic variant c.1771G > A was found to cause X-linked non-syndromic hearing loss DFNX6 with cochlear malformation in a Hungarian family [99].

4. Auditory neuropathy

Auditory Neuropathy was first defined by Arnold and his colleagues in 1996 while working on individuals with hearing loss. These individuals had normal outer hair cells in the cochlea, and preserved otoacoustic emissions while the ABRs were either absent or severely abnormal due to malfunction in eight cranial nerves. Auditory neuropathy may occur alone or as part of generalized neuropathic process [100].

Auditory neuropathy is divided into two categories according to the cause of neuropathy. In auditory neuropathy type I (AN type I) demyelination and axonal loss of auditory nerve is the predominant cause, while auditory neuropathy type II

(AN type II) occurs due to lesions in eight cranial nerves either at inner hair cells (IHCs) or synapses between IHCs and auditory nerve dendrites or at both [100–103].

Auditory neuropathy can be inherited as either non-syndromic or with accompanying clinical features as a syndrome. Syndromic auditory neuropathy can be due to dominant syndromes like Charcot-Marie-Tooth and Leber's Hereditary Optic Neuropathy (LHON) or recessive syndromes like Fredreich's Ataxia [104]. Mitochondrially inherited case of auditory neuropathy was reported by Deltenre et al. [105].

Non-syndromic auditory neuropathy can be dominant, recessive, or X-linked. AUNA1 was the first locus to be studied for autosomal dominant auditory neuropathy [106]. Pathogenic variants in *OTOF* cause non-syndromic recessive auditory neuropathy (NSRAN) [107]. Deafness due to *OTOF* gene variants is manifested in two ways:

1. non-syndromic auditory neuropathy spectrum disorder ANSD causing severe to profound bilateral deafness with congenital/prelingual onset.

2. temperature-sensitive auditory neuropathy spectrum disorder (TS-ANSD) with normal hearing at baseline body temperature and bilateral hearing loss on rising body temperature of 0.5°C or more with subsequent revival of hearing a few hours from achieving basal body temperature [108].

Some studies suggest variants in *GJB2* can cause non-syndromic recessive ANSD [109, 110]. X-linked pattern for NSRAN was identified when it was reported that *AUNX1* gene variant is responsible for causing auditory neuropathy and progressive peripheral sensory neuropathy in X- linked manner [111].

Since the discovery of auditory neuropathy scientists has been trying to pinpoint the underlying reason. A study has shown that more than 40% of cases of ANSD are due to hereditary neurological disorders [112]. Although majority of cases of ANSD are sporadic in nature, familial cases have also been reported [113].

The frequency of auditory neuropathy among patients with hearing loss has remained underestimated. In a recent study on Saudi Arabian children diagnosed with NSHL (non-syndromic hearing loss), 9.85% were identified to have ANSD [114]. Thus, the disorder is more prevalent than it was once thought. Other than genetic cause, one of the prominent reasons of auditory neuropathy is bilirubin toxicity, as it damages the auditory nerve and brainstem auditory nuclei [115].

5. Age-related hearing loss (ARHL)

Age-related hearing loss (ARHL) which is also known as presbycusis, is defined as a progressive, bilateral, and symmetrical sensorineural hearing loss which is mostly observed at high sound frequencies. It is the most common sensory deficit occurring in individuals over the age of 75, severely affecting their communication, cognitive abilities, and social activities [116]. ARHL is the third most prevalent health condition in the world, affecting older adults after heart disease and arthritis [117]. In estimation by the World Health Organization (WHO) 580 million people worldwide over the age of 65 are experiencing hearing loss. It is anticipated that by the next decade over one billion people over the age of 60 will be affected by ARHL (http://www.who.int/en/).

5.1 Etiology and classification

ARHL is a complex disorder which has both genetic and environmental causative factors [118]. In general, there are four major classes of ARHL each having a different cochlear biology and hearing phenotype. First type is the sensory presbycusis which is a progressive degeneration or loss of the inner and outer hair cells in cochlea. Individuals with sensory presbycusis usually have a steep sloping audiogram at high frequencies. The second type is the strial presbycusis which is characterized by the atrophy of stria vascularis. Individuals with strial presbycusis have relatively flat audiograms indicating loss of hearing over all the sound frequencies. Neural presbycusis is the third type which is defined by the degeneration of nerve fibers and patients with this type of pathology are unable to understand and distinguish speech. The fourth form of presbycusis is the cochlear-conductive or mechanical presbycusis which is caused by the changes in stiffness of basilar membrane in cochlea due to aging. Although microscopic findings are negligible in this type however, individuals exhibit gradual down sloping audiograms [119, 120].

5.2 Genetics of ARHL

Most people lose hearing acuity with age; however, it has been shown that genetic heritability also affects the susceptibility, time of onset, and severity of ARHL [118, 121, 122]. Although the biomolecular mechanisms of ARHL have been well defined but due to the complex pathology along with highly significant and variable environmental factors associated with ARHL, it has become difficult to identify the genetic contributors underlying ARHL. So far, researchers have investigated the genes involved in ARHL using familial and cohort-based approaches. However, genome wide association studies (GWAS), exome sequencing (ES) and genome sequencing (GS) on large cohorts have been more helpful revealing the genetic susceptibilities underlying ARHL. There are variants and Single Neucleotide Polymorphisms (SNPs) in more than 15 genes which are found responsible and have been well-studied for presbycusis in human or mouse models. In addition, ultra-rare heterozygous variants of known deafness genes have also been shown to cause severe form of ARHL [123].

Following is the detail of these genes which account for ARHL studied in different populations.

5.3 Genes involved in membrane transport and cellular adhesion

5.3.1 Solute carrier family 12 member 2 (SLC12A2)

SLC12A2 also referred to as $Na^+K^+2xCl^-$ co-transporter (NKCC1) is a member of solute carrier family 12 which is involved in the transport of sodium, potassium, and chloride ions across the secretory and absorptive epithelia [124]. It is found to be expressed in the basolateral membrane of marginal strial cells and in the lateral wall fibrocytes in cochlea of rodents and non-human primates. Fibrocytes take up K^+ from perilymph through SLC12A2 and ATP1A2 (α2-Na^+K^+ATPase) [125, 126] and pass it to intermediate cells and strial basal cells through gap junctions [127]. It also transports K^+ from the intra-strial space into the marginal cells [128]. In mice, it has been shown that heterozygous variants in *Slc12a2* can result in progressive ARHL without causing any damage to the cochlear morphology [129]. However, the role of this gene for ARHL in humans has not been tested yet.

5.3.2 Voltage gated potassium channel KQT like subfamily member 4 (KCNQ4)

Potassium channels play an important role in maintaining ionic composition and electrical signaling in biological fluids. Cochlear hair cells and vestibular structures have voltage-gated potassium channels encoded by *KCNQ4* to maintain ionic balance in cochlear fluid [130]. Missense variants in *KCNQ4* are commonly known to cause non-syndromic autosomal dominant hearing loss, DFNA2 [131–134]. However, in a study of two Caucasian populations, several SNPs were found associated with ARHL, all of which were localized to a 13 kb region in the middle of the *KCNQ4* [135].

5.3.3 Wolframin (WFS1)

WFS1 encodes Wolframin which is a transmembrane protein and is thought to be a large cation-selective ion channel [136]. Variants in *WFS1* commonly cause Wolfram syndrome [137], and non-syndromic autosomal dominant low frequency sensorineural hearing loss [138–140]. In 2017, a study comprising 518 Finnish adults showed a heterozygous variant p.(Tyr528His) associated with late-onset hearing loss. Most of the individuals participating in this cohort initially had hearing loss which affected the high frequencies and subsequently progressed to involve middle and low frequencies [141].

5.3.4 Solute carrier family 7 member 8 (SLC7A8)

SLC7A8 functions as a sodium-independent transporter of L-type amino acids in many organs in vertebrates [142]. It is highly expressed in the inner ear [143, 144], and specifically localizes to the stria vascularis [143]. A study focused on the role of *Slc7a8* in ARHL using mouse models demonstrated that in homozygous knockout mice (*Slc7a8*$^{-/-}$) the loss of function leads to high-frequency hearing loss which progressively extends to low frequencies. While, interestingly, the young knockout mice heterozygous for *Slc7a8* (*Slc7a8*$^{+/-}$) did not show a hearing loss. However, with aging, these mice developed high-frequency hearing loss earlier than the wild-type mice [144]. Similarly, in a cohort of 66 ARHL patients from Italy, genome sequencing identified four heterozygous variants (p.Val302Ile, p.Arg418His, p.Thr402Met and p.Val460Glu) in SLC7A8 [144]. In vitro functional studies of these variants further confirmed a significant decrease in amino acid transport activity supporting *SLC7A8* as a causative gene for ARHL.

5.4 Mitochondrial antioxidative enzymes

Mitochondrial DNA (mtDNA) variants have long been known to cause various human diseases, including non-syndromic hearing loss [145]. A significant increase in the contribution of mtDNA variants has been observed in aging human auditory system [146]. The postmortem analyses of human temporal bones have shown a 4977 bp deletion (also known as common deletion (CD)) in mtDNA as a frequent cause of ARHL [147, 148]. Additionally, a decrease in the expression of another mitochondrial enzyme cytochrome oxidase 3 (*COX3*) in spiral ganglion cells was also reported in ARHL patients [149].

Isocitrate dehydrogenase (*IDH*) is a key component of the aerobic metabolism in mitochondria, which facilitates the generation of NADPH and NADH thus regulating the cellular oxidative stress [150, 151]. It has been demonstrated in a mouse study that the expression of *IDH2* normally decreases with age and when this gene was knocked out there was increased oxidative stress in the murine inner ear leading to the loss of hair cells and damage to spiral ganglion [152].

5.5 Hormonal factors

5.5.1 Insulin like growth factor 1 (IGF1)

Animal studies suggest that *Igf1* promotes inner ear neuronal development by supporting neurogenesis, differentiation, and proliferation of neuronal progenitor cells [153, 154]. It has been ubiquitously detected in mouse inner ear, including the spiral ganglion, spiral ligament, stria vascularis, hair cells, and vestibular tissues [155–157]. Numerous variants in *IGF1* have been associated with sensorineural hearing loss in humans and Larson's syndrome; patients who also suffer from early-onset ARHL [158–160].

5.5.2 Estrogen related receptor γ (*ESRRG*)

Esrrg mRNA has been shown to be expressed at embryonic stages in the mouse cochlear and vestibular ganglion [161], which suggests a role in the inner ear function and development. Moreover, there is considerable evidence supporting an auditory protective effect of estrogen and estrogen-related receptors on the auditory system [162, 163]. In humans, several studies have shown that ARHL is more common and severe with early onset in men as compared to women [164, 165]. For instance, in an analysis of 6134 individuals from three separate European cohorts, an association was found between the minor allele of SNP *rs2818964* and hearing status only in women. Additionally, *Esrrg* knockout mice revealed that at 12 weeks, average hearing thresholds in female mice were 15 dB worse than in males [166].

5.6 Genes involved in metabolic pathways

Studies on human subjects with ARHL have also identified specific polymorphisms in a few genes involved in the folate metabolism pathway. A recent report that genotyped an ARHL cohort from South India revealed several specific polymorphisms within genes encoding thymidylate synthase (*TYMS*) and 5,10-methylenetetrahydrofolate reductase (*MTHFR*). Some polymorphisms such as the *MTHFR* A1298C were noted to protect against the development of ARHL, while others such as *MTHFR* C677T were associated with an increased risk of ARHL in this population [167].

5.7 Other genes identified for ARHL

5.7.1 Glutamate receptor metabotropic 7 (GRM7)

GRM7 encodes a G-protein coupled receptor which plays an important role in the regulation of presynaptic neurotransmission in the mammalian brain. It is widely expressed in inner hair cells, outer hair cells, spiral ganglion, and vestibular hair cells. The expression of this gene increases with age [168]. GWAS on 3434 well-characterized individuals from different locations in Europe identified SNPs in *GRM7* causing ARHL [168]. Two more studies on an American and Saami population cohort also corroborated the potential role of *GRM7* in ARHL [169, 170].

5.7.2 Grainyhead drosophila homolog of 2 (GRHL2)

GRHL2 is known to have an essential role in the development and morphogenesis of epithelia of several organs in flies, mice, frogs, and zebrafish [171]. Variants in *GRHL2* have been known to cause non-syndromic autosomal dominant hearing loss [172, 173]. Additionally, a study comprised of 2418 cases from seven different European countries emphasized the association of SNPs enriched in intron 1 of *GRHL2* with ARHL [174].

5.7.3 Neuropillin-1 (Nrp1)

NRP1 is an essential component of Neurolippin-1/Semaphorin 3A signaling pathway. This pathway is responsible for the proper development of vascular and neuronal structures in inner ear as well as hair cell organization [175, 176]. A GWAS study on mice showed progressive hearing loss with age and abnormalities in inner ear microvasculature [177]. Although these investigations suggest that *Nrp1* can be associated with ARHL in mice, no such studies have been performed in humans.

5.7.4 Cadherin related family member 23 ($Cdh23^{Ahl}$)

$Cdh23^{\mathrm{Ahl}}$ is characterized as a hypomorphic allele for a calcium-dependent cell adhesion protein, otocadherin. It helps in the organization of stereocilia bundle and vestibular hair cells and is required for maintaining this organization in later stages of life [178]. Based on the association of $Cdh23^{\mathrm{Ahl}}$ with ARHL in mice, GWAS on a large cohort of Han Chinese population was performed to investigate the role of *CDH23* in ARHL in humans. This study demonstrated that SNPs in *CDH23* do not cause ARHL in humans [179]. However, another study on the methylation patterns in *CDH23* showed a positive correlation between an increase in methylation of the gene and ARHL [180].

6. Tinnitus

Tinnitus is derived from a Latin verb tinnire (to ring), and it describes the conscious perception of hissing, sizzling, or ringing sound in the absence of a corresponding external stimulus. Tinnitus can sometimes be random voices, music, or a mixture of sounds [181]. It can be constant or intermittent, or may be perceived in one (mostly left) or both ears, or centrally within the head. The reason for the left-sided predisposition of tinnitus is yet unknown.

Most of the studies to investigate the prevalence of tinnitus have been carried out in USA or Europe which gave a rough estimate of 10–15% of individuals suffering from tinnitus in these populations. National Study of Hearing in England was one of the largest (n = 48,313) and most reliable studies conducted to determine the prevalence of tinnitus among adult population. The results showed a prevalence of 10–15% among adults. Similarly, results from studies in Egypt [182, 183], Japan [184–186], and Nigeria [187, 188], also indicated that the rate of prevalence of tinnitus in these countries is analogous to the results from the Europe [189] and the USA [190–192].

6.1 Risk factors and genetic pathology of tinnitus

There are many risk factors known to be associated with tinnitus. To name one of the most common is hearing loss. All the patients with hearing loss may not develop tinnitus, however, individuals with tinnitus have a predictive diagnosis for hearing loss depending on the responses to pure tone thresholds [181]. Other possible risk factors include noise exposure, head trauma, obesity, alcohol consumption, and ototoxic drugs, such as salicylates, quinines and platinum-based drugs can also trigger tinnitus. It can also be found associated with severe otological diseases like Meinnere's disease, acoustic neuroma, and otosclerosis [193].

There are many publications stating the risk factors for tinnitus, but none of them describes the complete mechanism or molecular biology of this disorder. It is speculated that tinnitus is also caused by cochlear or auditory nerve damage. Despite its close relatedness to hearing loss patients suffering from tinnitus do not have the auditory nerve or cochlear degeneration as a common cause. This indicates the involvement of other systems in the brain with or without the involvement of the auditory system.

Determination of heritability of tinnitus remained an important task and it is still an arguable debate in the field. A large study held in Norway shows a significant familial aggregation of tinnitus among the participating population (aged >75 years) [194]. There are few more studies that emphasize the involvement of genetic factors in tinnitus with slight variation in their data [195]. The variation in the results may have appeared due to small sample size or the difference in population characteristics. With the utilization of new scientific technologies, it can be expected that researchers will provide a better and more appropriate conclusion to this debate.

7. Conclusion

Hearing loss is one of the most common sensory defects that affects about 5% of the world population. Genetics is a major contributor to deafness causing about 50% of all cases. Although elucidation of the genetics of hearing loss has advanced rapidly in the past 20 years, still lacking is a complete understanding of all the networks and pathways required for normal audition. In future, continued studies will reveal further insights into function of the auditory system and treatment due to its malfunction.

Author details

Hina Khan[1,†], Hafiza Idrees[2,†], Zunaira Munir[3*] and Memoona Ramzan[4*]

1 School of Biological Sciences, University of the Punjab, Lahore, Pakistan

2 Experimental Cardiology, Justus Liebig University Giessen, Germany

3 Department of Neuroscience, University of Turin, Turin, Italy

4 Dr. John T. Macdonald Foundation Department of Human Genetics and John P. Hussman Institute for Human Genetics, University of Miami, Miller School of Medicine, Miami, FL, USA

*Address all correspondence to: zunaira.munir@unito.it; mxr2595@med.miami.edu

† Hina Khan and Hafiza Idrees are co-first authors.

References

[1] Nadol JB. Hearing loss. New England Journal of Medicine. 1993;**329**(15):1092-1102

[2] Anastasiadou S, Al Khalili Y. Hearing Loss. Treasure Island (FL): StatPearls Publishing; 2021

[3] Steel KP. New interventions in hearing impairment. BMJ. 2000;**320**(7235):622-625

[4] Richard EM, Santos-Cortez RLP, Faridi R, Rehman AU, Lee K, Shahzad M, et al. Global genetic insight contributed by consanguineous Pakistani families segregating hearing loss. Human Mutation. 2019;**40**(1):53-72

[5] Yamasoba T, Lin FR, Someya S, Kashio A, Sakamoto T, Kondo K. Current concepts in age-related hearing loss: Epidemiology and mechanistic pathways. Hearing Research. 2013;**303**:30-38

[6] Davis AC, Hoffman HJ. Hearing loss: Rising prevalence and impact. Bulletin of the World Health Organization. 2019;**97**(10):646

[7] Smith RJ, Bale JF Jr, White KR. Sensorineural hearing loss in children. The Lancet. 2005;**365**(9462):879-890

[8] Hilgert N, Smith RJ, Van Camp G. Forty-six genes causing nonsyndromic hearing impairment: Which ones should be analyzed in DNA diagnostics? Mutation Research/Reviews in Mutation Research. 2009;**681**(2-3):189-196

[9] Kochhar A, Hildebrand MS, Smith RJ. Clinical aspects of hereditary hearing loss. Genetics in Medicine. 2007;**9**(7):393

[10] Panel GEoCHLE: Genetics evaluation guidelines for the etiologic diagnosis of congenital hearing loss. Genetics in Medicine. 2002;**4**(3):162

[11] Bayazit YA, Yilmaz M. An overview of hereditary hearing loss. ORL; Journal for Oto-rhino-laryngology and its Related Specialties. 2006;**68**(2):57-63

[12] Duman D, Tekin M. Autosomal recessive nonsyndromic deafness genes: A review. Frontiers in Bioscience: A Journal and Virtual Library. 2012;**17**:2213

[13] Shafique S, Siddiqi S, Schraders M, Oostrik J, Ayub H, Bilal A, et al. Genetic spectrum of autosomal recessive non-syndromic hearing loss in Pakistani families. PLoS One. 2014;**9**(6):e100146

[14] Hone SW, Smith RJ. Genetic screening for hearing loss. Clinical Otolaryngology & Allied Sciences. 2003;**28**(4):285-290

[15] Skvorak AG, Morton CC. Genetic causes of nonsyndromic hearing loss. Current Opinion in Pediatrics. 1999;**11**(6):551-557

[16] Friedman TB, Griffith AJ. Human nonsyndromic sensorineural deafness. Annual Review of Genomics and Human Genetics. 2003;**4**(1):341-402

[17] Parker M, Bitner-Glindzicz M. Genetic investigations in childhood deafness. Archives of Disease in Childhood. 2015;**100**(3):271-278

[18] Stelma F, Bhutta MF. Non-syndromic hereditary sensorineural hearing loss: Review of the genes involved. The Journal of Laryngology and Otology. 2014;**128**(1):13-21

[19] Babanejad M, Beheshtian M, Jamshidi F, Mohseni M, Booth KT,

Kahrizi K, et al. Genetic etiology of hearing loss in Iran. Human Genetics. 2022;**141**:623-631

[20] Anwar S, Riazuddin S, Ahmed ZM, Tasneem S, Ateeq ul J, Khan SY, et al. SLC26A4 mutation spectrum associated with DFNB4 deafness and Pendred's syndrome in Pakistanis. Journal of Human Genetics. 2009;**54**(5):266-270

[21] Bizhanova A, Kopp P. Genetics and phenomics of Pendred syndrome. Molecular and Cellular Endocrinology. 2010;**322**(1):83-90

[22] Wémeau JL, Kopp P. Pendred syndrome. Best Practice & Research Clinical Endocrinology & Metabolism. 2017;**31**(2):213-224

[23] Honda K, Griffith A. Genetic architecture and phenotypic landscape of SLC26A4-related hearing loss. Human Genetics. 2021;**141**:455-464

[24] Choi BY, Stewart AK, Madeo AC, Pryor SP, Lenhard S, Kittles R, et al. Hypo-functional SLC26A4 variants associated with nonsyndromic hearing loss and enlargement of the vestibular aqueduct: Genotype-phenotype correlation or coincidental polymorphisms? Human Mutation. 2009;**30**(4):599-608

[25] Tsukamoto K, Suzuki H, Harada D, Namba A, Abe S, Usami S-I. Distribution and frequencies of PDS (SLC26A4) mutations in Pendred syndrome and nonsyndromic hearing loss associated with enlarged vestibular aqueduct: A unique spectrum of mutations in Japanese. European Journal of Human Genetics. 2003;**11**(12):916-922

[26] Ouyang XM, Yan D, Du LL, Hejtmancik JF, Jacobson SG, Nance WE, et al. Characterization of Usher syndrome type I gene mutations in an Usher syndrome patient population. Human Genetics. 2005;**116**(4):292-299

[27] Millán JM, Aller E, Jaijo T, Blanco-Kelly F, Gimenez-Pardo A, Ayuso C. An update on the genetics of Usher syndrome. Journal of Ophthalmology. 2011;**2011**:417217

[28] Castiglione A, Möller C. Usher syndrome. Audiology Research. 2022;**12**(1):42-65

[29] Mathur P, Yang J. Usher syndrome: Hearing loss, retinal degeneration and associated abnormalities. Biochimica et Biophysica Acta. 2015;**1852**(3):406-420

[30] Pingault V, Faubert E, Baral V, Gherbi S, Loundon N, Couloigner V, et al. SOX10 mutations mimic isolated hearing loss. Clinical Genetics. 2014;**88**:352-359

[31] Bademci G, Cengiz FB, Foster Ii J, Duman D, Sennaroglu L, Diaz-Horta O, et al. Variations in multiple syndromic deafness genes mimic non-syndromic hearing loss. Scientific Reports. 2016;**6**(1):31622

[32] Bolz HJ. Hereditary hearing loss and its syndromes third edition. European Journal of Human Genetics. 2016;**24**(11):1650-1650

[33] Petersen M, Willems P. Non-syndromic, autosomal-recessive deafness. Clinical Genetics. 2006;**69**(5):371-392

[34] Van Camp GSR. Hereditary Hearing Loss Homepage. 2022. Available from: https://hereditaryhearinglossorg

[35] Hilgert N, Smith RJH, Van Camp G. Forty-six genes causing nonsyndromic hearing impairment: Which ones should be analyzed in DNA diagnostics? Mutation Research. 2009;**681**(2-3):189-196

[36] Guilford P, Arab SB, Blanchard S, Levilliers J, Weissenbach J, Belkahia A, et al. A non-syndromic form of neurosensory, recessive deafness maps to the pericentromeric region of chromosome 13q. Nature Genetics. 1994;**6**(1):24-28

[37] Kelsell DP, Dunlop J, Stevens HP, Lench NJ, Liang JN, Parry G, et al. Connexin 26 mutations in hereditary non-syndromic sensorineural deafness. Nature. 1997;**387**(6628):80-83

[38] Kelley PM, Harris DJ, Comer BC, Askew JW, Fowler T, Smith SD, et al. Novel mutations in the connexin 26 gene (GJB2) that cause autosomal recessive (DFNB1) hearing loss. American Journal of Human Genetics. 1998;**62**(4):792-799

[39] Qu Y, Tang W, Zhou B, Ahmad S, Chang Q, Li X, et al. Early developmental expression of connexin26 in the cochlea contributes to its dominate functional role in the cochlear gap junctions. Biochemical and Biophysical Research Communications. 2012;**417**(1):245-250

[40] Koohiyan M, Koohian F, Azadegan-Dehkordi F. GJB2-related hearing loss in Central Iran: Review of the spectrum and frequency of gene mutations. Annals of Human Genetics. 2020;**84**(2):107-113

[41] Santos RLP, Wajid M, Pham TL, Hussan J, Ali G, Ahmad W, et al. Low prevalence of Connexin 26 (GJB2) variants in Pakistani families with autosomal recessive non-syndromic hearing impairment. Clinical Genetics. 2005;**67**(1):61-68

[42] Salman M, Bashir R, Imtiaz A, Maqsood A, Mujtaba G, Iqbal M, et al. Mutations of GJB2 encoding connexin 26 contribute to non-syndromic moderate and severe hearing loss in Pakistan. European Archives of Oto-rhino-laryngology: Official Journal of the European Federation of Oto-Rhino-Laryngological Societies (EUFOS): Affiliated with the German Society for Oto-Rhino-Laryngology—Head and Neck Surgery. 2015;**272**(8):2071-2075

[43] Chan DK, Chang KW. GJB2-associated hearing loss: Systematic review of worldwide prevalence, genotype, and auditory phenotype. The Laryngoscope. 2014;**124**(2):E34-E53

[44] Everett LA, Glaser B, Beck JC, Idol JR, Buchs A, Ma H, et al. Pendred syndrome is caused by mutations in a putative sulphate transporter gene (PDS). Nature Genetics. 1997;**17**(4):411-422

[45] Li XC, Everett LA, Lalwani AK, Desmukh D, Friedman TB, Green ED, et al. A mutation in PDS causes non-syndromic recessive deafness. Nature Genetics. 1998;**18**(3):215-217

[46] Wémeau J-L, Kopp P. Pendred syndrome. Best Practice & Research Clinical Endocrinology & Metabolism. 2017;**31**(2):213-224

[47] Everett LA, Belyantseva IA, Noben-Trauth K, Cantos R, Chen A, Thakkar SI, et al. Targeted disruption of mouse Pds provides insight about the inner-ear defects encountered in Pendred syndrome. Human Molecular Genetics. 2001;**10**(2):153-161

[48] Nakaya K, Harbidge DG, Wangemann P, Schultz BD, Green ED, Wall SM, et al. Lack of pendrin HCO3– transport elevates vestibular endolymphatic [Ca2+] by inhibition of acid-sensitive TRPV5 and TRPV6 channels. American Journal of Physiology-Renal Physiology. 2007;**292**(5):F1314-F1321

[49] Yang T, Gurrola JG 2nd, Wu H, Chiu SM, Wangemann P, Snyder PM,

et al. Mutations of KCNJ10 together with mutations of SLC26A4 cause digenic nonsyndromic hearing loss associated with enlarged vestibular aqueduct syndrome. American Journal of Human Genetics. 2009;**84**(5):651-657

[50] Li M, Nishio S-Y, Naruse C, Riddell M, Sapski S, Katsuno T, et al. Digenic inheritance of mutations in EPHA2 and SLC26A4 in Pendred syndrome. Nature Communications. 2020;**11**(1):1343-1343

[51] Wang A, Liang Y, Fridell RA, Probst FJ, Wilcox ER, Touchman JW, et al. Association of unconventional myosin *MYO15* mutations with human nonsyndromic deafness *DFNB3*. Science. 1998;**280**(5368):1447-1451

[52] Friedman TB, Liang Y, Weber JL, Hinnant JT, Barber TD, Winata S, et al. A gene for congenital, recessive deafness DFNB3 maps to the pericentromeric region of chromosome 17. Nature Genetics. 1995;**9**(1):86-91

[53] Liang Y, Wang A, Belyantseva IA, Anderson DW, Probst FJ, Barber TD, et al. Characterization of the human and mouse unconventional myosin XV genes responsible for hereditary deafness DFNB3 and shaker 2. Genomics. 1999;**61**(3):243-258

[54] Weck ML, Grega-Larson NE, Tyska MJ. MyTH4-FERM myosins in the assembly and maintenance of actin-based protrusions. Current Opinion in Cell Biology. 2017;**44**:68-78

[55] Du H, Li N, Xu Z. Myosin XVA: Dancing at the tips of the stereocilia. Journal of Bio-X Research. 2020;**03**(02):60-65

[56] Zhang J, Guan J, Wang H, Yin L, Wang D, Zhao L, et al. Genotype-phenotype correlation analysis of MYO15A variants in autosomal recessive non-syndromic hearing loss. BMC Medical Genetics. 2019;**20**(1):60-60

[57] Fattahi Z, Shearer AE, Babanejad M, Bazazzadegan N, Almadani SN, Nikzat N, et al. Screening for MYO15A gene mutations in autosomal recessive nonsyndromic, GJB2 negative Iranian deaf population. American Journal of Medical Genetics Part A. 2012;**158A**(8):1857-1864

[58] Han JJ, Nguyen PD, Oh D-Y, Han JH, Kim A-R, Kim MY, et al. Elucidation of the unique mutation spectrum of severe hearing loss in a Vietnamese pediatric population. Scientific Reports. 2019;**9**(1):1604

[59] Si Y, Grati M, Cohen-Salmon M, El-Amraoui A, Mustapha M, Salem N, et al. A mutation in OTOF, encoding otoferlin, a FER-1-like protein, causes DFNB9, a nonsyndromic form of deafness. Nature Genetics. 1999;**21**(4):363-369

[60] Roux I, Safieddine S, Nouvian R, Grati M, Simmler M-C, Bahloul A, et al. Otoferlin, defective in a human deafness form, is essential for exocytosis at the auditory ribbon synapse. Cell. 2006;**127**(2):277-289

[61] Mahdieh N, Shirkavand A, Rabbani B, Tekin M, Akbari B, Akbari MT, et al. Screening of OTOF mutations in Iran: A novel mutation and review. International Journal of Pediatric Otorhinolaryngology. 2012;**76**(11):1610-1615

[62] Doyle KJ, Sininger Y, Starr A. Auditory neuropathy in childhood. The Laryngoscope. 1998;**108**(9):1374-1377

[63] Zheng D, Liu X. Cochlear implantation outcomes in patients with OTOF mutations. Frontiers in Neuroscience. 2020;**14**:1-7

[64] Bolz H, von Brederlow B, Ramírez A, Bryda EC, Kutsche K, Nothwang HG, et al. Mutation of CDH23, encoding a new member of the cadherin gene family, causes Usher syndrome type 1D. Nature Genetics. 2001;**27**(1):108-112

[65] Kazmierczak P, Sakaguchi H, Tokita J, Wilson-Kubalek EM, Milligan RA, Müller U, et al. Cadherin 23 and protocadherin 15 interact to form tip-link filaments in sensory hair cells. Nature. 2007;**449**(7158):87-91

[66] Schultz JM, Bhatti R, Madeo AC, Turriff A, Muskett JA, Zalewski CK, et al. Allelic hierarchy of CDH23 mutations causing non-syndromic deafness DFNB12 or Usher syndrome USH1D in compound heterozygotes. Journal of Medical Genetics. 2011;**48**(11):767-775

[67] Chen K, Huang B, Sun J, Liang Y, Xiong G. Cochlear implantation outcomes in children with CDH23 mutations-associated hearing loss. Otolaryngology—Head and Neck Surgery: Official Journal of American Academy of Otolaryngology-Head and Neck Surgery. 2021;**1945998211057427**

[68] Kurima K, Peters LM, Yang Y, Riazuddin S, Ahmed ZM, Naz S, et al. Dominant and recessive deafness caused by mutations of a novel gene, TMC1, required for cochlear hair-cell function. Nature Genetics. 2002;**30**(3):277-284

[69] Pan B, Akyuz N, Liu X-P, Asai Y, Nist-Lund C, Kurima K, et al. TMC1 forms the pore of Mechanosensory transduction channels in vertebrate inner ear hair cells. Neuron. 2018;**99**(4): 736-753.e736

[70] Kitajiri S-i, McNamara R, Makishima T, Husnain T, Zafar A, Kittles R, et al. Identities, frequencies and origins of TMC1 mutations causing DFNB7/B11 deafness in Pakistan. Clinical Genetics. 2007;**72**(6):546-550

[71] Sommen M, Schrauwen I, Vandeweyer G, Boeckx N, Corneveaux JJ, van den Ende J, et al. DNA diagnostics of hereditary hearing loss: A targeted resequencing approach combined with a mutation classification system. Human Mutation. 2016;**37**(8):812-819

[72] Kalay E, Karaguzel A, Caylan R, Heister A, Cremers FP, Cremers CW, et al. Four novel TMC1 (DFNB7/ DFNB11) mutations in Turkish patients with congenital autosomal recessive nonsyndromic hearing loss. Human Mutation. 2005;**26**(6):591

[73] Sırmacı A, Duman D, Öztürkmen-Akay H, Erbek S, İncesulu A, Öztürk-Hişmi B, et al. Mutations in TMC1 contribute significantly to nonsyndromic autosomal recessive sensorineural hearing loss: A report of five novel mutations. International Journal of Pediatric Otorhinolaryngology. 2009;**73**(5):699-705

[74] Naz S. Molecular genetic landscape of hereditary hearing loss in Pakistan. Human Genetics. 2021;**141**:633-648

[75] Richard EM, Santos-Cortez RLP, Faridi R, Rehman AU, Lee K, Shahzad M, et al. Global genetic insight contributed by consanguineous Pakistani families segregating hearing loss. Human Mutation. 2019;**40**(1):53-72

[76] Schultz JM, Khan SN, Ahmed ZM, Riazuddin S, Waryah AM, Chhatre D, et al. Noncoding mutations of HGF are associated with nonsyndromic hearing loss, DFNB39. American Journal of Human Genetics. 2009;**85**(1):25-39

[77] Ma Y, Xiao Y, Zhang F, Han Y, Li J, Xu L, et al. Novel compound heterozygous mutations in MYO7A gene associated with autosomal recessive sensorineural hearing loss in a Chinese family. International Journal of Pediatric Otorhinolaryngology. 2016;**83**:179-185

[78] Liu XZ, Walsh J, Tamagawa Y, Kitamura K, Nishizawa M, Steel KP, et al. Autosomal dominant non-syndromic deafness caused by a mutation in the myosin VIIA gene. Nature Genetics. 1997;**17**(3):268-269

[79] Tang P-C, Alex A, Nie J, Lee J, Roth A, Booth K, et al. Defective Tmprss3-associated hair cell degeneration in inner ear organoids. Stem Cell Reports. 2019;**13**:147-162

[80] Gao X, Huang SS, Yuan YY, Xu JC, Gu P, Bai D, et al. Identification of TMPRSS3 as a significant contributor to autosomal recessive hearing loss in the Chinese population. Neural Plasticity. 2017;**2017**:3192090

[81] Guipponi M, Vuagniaux G, Wattenhofer M, Shibuya K, Vazquez M, Dougherty L, et al. The transmembrane serine protease (TMPRSS3) mutated in deafness DFNB8/10 activates the epithelial sodium channel (ENaC) in vitro. Human Molecular Genetics. 2002;**11**(23):2829-2836

[82] Lee YJ, Park D, Kim SY, Park WJ. Pathogenic mutations but not polymorphisms in congenital and childhood onset autosomal recessive deafness disrupt the proteolytic activity of TMPRSS3. Journal of Medical Genetics. 2003;**40**(8):629-631

[83] Molina L, Fasquelle L, Nouvian R, Salvetat N, Scott HS, Guipponi M, et al. Tmprss3 loss of function impairs cochlear inner hair cell Kcnma1 channel membrane expression. Human Molecular Genetics. 2013;**22**(7):1289-1299

[84] Kubisch C, Schroeder BC, Friedrich T, Lütjohann B, El-Amraoui A, Marlin S, et al. KCNQ4, a novel potassium channel expressed in sensory outer hair cells, is mutated in dominant deafness. Cell. 1999;**96**(3):437-446

[85] Ramzan M, Idrees H, Mujtaba G, Sobreira N, Witmer PD, Naz S. Bi-allelic Pro291Leu variant in KCNQ4 leads to early onset non-syndromic hearing loss. Gene. 2019;**705**:109-112

[86] Wasano K, Mutai H, Obuchi C, Masuda S, Matsunaga T. A novel frameshift mutation in KCNQ4 in a family with autosomal recessive non-syndromic hearing loss. Biochemical and Biophysical Research Communications. 2015;**463**(4):582-586

[87] Kojima T, Wasano K, Takahashi S, Homma K. Cell death-inducing cytotoxicity in truncated KCNQ4 variants associated with DFNA2 hearing loss. Disease Models & Mechanisms. 2021;**11**:1-12

[88] Peixoto Pinheiro B, Vona B, Löwenheim H, Rüttiger L, Knipper M, Adel Y. Age-related hearing loss pertaining to potassium ion channels in the cochlea and auditory pathway. Pflugers Archiv: European Journal of Physiology. 2021;**473**(5):823-840

[89] Robertson NG, Lu L, Heller S, Merchant SN, Eavey RD, McKenna M, et al. Mutations in a novel cochlear gene cause DFNA9, a human nonsyndromic deafness with vestibular dysfunction. Nature Genetics. 1998;**20**(3):299-303

[90] Robertson NG, O'Malley JT, Ong CA, Giersch ABS, Shen J, Stankovic KM, et al. Cochlin in normal middle ear and abnormal middle ear deposits in DFNA9 and Coch (G88E/G88E) mice. Journal of the Association for Research in Otolaryngology. 2014;**15**(6):961-974

[91] JanssensdeVarebeke SPF, Van Camp G, Peeters N, Elinck E, Widdershoven J, Cox T, et al. Bi-allelic inactivating variants in the COCH gene cause autosomal recessive prelingual hearing impairment. European Journal of Human Genetics. 2018;**26**(4):587-591

[92] Strom TM, Hörtnagel K, Hofmann S, Gekeler F, Scharfe C, Rabl W, et al. Diabetes insipidus, diabetes mellitus, optic atrophy and deafness (DIDMOAD) caused by mutations in a novel gene (Wolframin) coding for a predicted transmembrane protein. Human Molecular Genetics. 1998;7(13):2021-2028

[93] Bespalova IN, Van Camp G, Bom SJ, Brown DJ, Cryns K, DeWan AT, et al. Mutations in the Wolfram syndrome 1 gene (WFS1) are a common cause of low frequency sensorineural hearing loss. Human Molecular Genetics. 2001;**10**(22):2501-2508

[94] Richard G, White TW, Smith LE, Bailey RA, Compton JG, Paul DL, et al. Functional defects of Cx26 resulting from a heterozygous missense mutation in a family with dominant deaf-mutism and palmoplantar keratoderma. Human Genetics. 1998;**103**(4):393-399

[95] Löffler J, Nekahm D, Hirst-Stadlmann A, Günther B, Menzel H-J, Utermann G, et al. Sensorineural hearing loss and the incidence of Cx26 mutations in Austria. European Journal of Human Genetics. 2001;**9**(3):226-230

[96] Liu X, Han D, Li J, Han B, Ouyang X, Cheng J, et al. Loss-of-function mutations in the PRPS1 gene cause a type of nonsyndromic X-linked sensorineural deafness, DFN2. American Journal of Human Genetics. 2010;**86**(1):65-71

[97] Huebner Antje K, Gandia M, Frommolt P, Maak A, Wicklein Eva M, Thiele H, et al. Nonsense mutations in SMPX, encoding a protein responsive to physical force, result in X-chromosomal hearing loss. The American Journal of Human Genetics. 2011;**88**(5):621-627

[98] Zong L, Guan J, Ealy M, Zhang Q, Wang D, Wang H, et al. Mutations in apoptosis-inducing factor cause X-linked recessive auditory neuropathy spectrum disorder. Journal of Medical Genetics. 2015;**52**(8):523-531

[99] Rost S, Bach E, Neuner C, Nanda I, Dysek S, Bittner RE, et al. Novel form of X-linked nonsyndromic hearing loss with cochlear malformation caused by a mutation in the type IV collagen gene COL4A6. European Journal of Human Genetics: EJHG. 2014;**22**(2):208-215

[100] Starr A, Picton TW, Sininger Y, Hood LJ, Berlin CI. Auditory neuropathy. Brain. 1996;**119**(3):741-753

[101] Bonfils P, Avan P, Londero A, Narcy P, Trotoux J. Progressive hereditary deafness with predominant inner hair cell loss. The American Journal of Otology. 1991;**12**(3):203-206

[102] Berlin CI. Auditory neuropathy. Current Opinion in Otolaryngology & Head and Neck Surgery. 1998;**6**(5)

[103] Leonardis L, Zidar J, Popovič M, Timmerman V, Löfgren A, Broeckhoven CV, et al. Hereditary motor and sensory neuropathy associated with auditory neuropathy in a Gypsy family. Pflügers Archiv. 2000;**439**(1):r208-r210

[104] Manchaiah VK, Zhao F, Danesh AA, Duprey R. The genetic basis of auditory neuropathy spectrum disorder (ANSD). International Journal of Pediatric Otorhinolaryngology. 2011;**75**(2):151-158

[105] Deltenre P, Mansbach AL, Bozet C, Clercx A, Hecox KE. Auditory neuropathy: A report on three cases with early onsets and major neonatal illnesses. Electroencephalography and Clinical Neurophysiology. 1997;**104**(1):17-22

[106] Kim TB, Isaacson B, Sivakumaran TA, Starr A, Keats BJ, Lesperance MM. A gene responsible

for autosomal dominant auditory neuropathy (AUNA1) maps to 13q14-21. Journal of Medical Genetics. 2004;**41**(11):872-876

[107] Varga R, Kelley PM, Keats BJ, Starr A, Leal SM, Cohn E, et al. Non-syndromic recessive auditory neuropathy is the result of mutations in the otoferlin (OTOF) gene. Journal of Medical Genetics. 2003;**40**(1):45-50

[108] Azaiez H, Thorpe RK, Smith RJH. OTOF-related deafness. In: Adam MP, Ardinger HH, Pagon RA, Wallace SE, LJH B, Gripp KW, Mirzaa GM, Amemiya A, editors. GeneReviews(®). Seattle (WA): University of Washington, Seattle; 1993

[109] Cheng X, Li L, Brashears S, Morlet T, Ng SS, Berlin C, et al. Connexin 26 variants and auditory neuropathy/dys-synchrony among children in schools for the deaf. American Journal of Medical Genetics Part A. 2005;**139**(1):13-18

[110] Santarelli R, Cama E, Scimemi P, Dal Monte E, Genovese E, Arslan E. Audiological and electrocochleography findings in hearing-impaired children with connexin 26 mutations and otoacoustic emissions. European Archives of Oto-rhino-laryngology: Official Journal of the European Federation of Oto-Rhino-Laryngological Societies (EUFOS): Affiliated with the German Society for Oto-Rhino-Laryngology—Head and Neck Surgery. 2008;**265**(1):43-51

[111] Wang QJ, Li QZ, Rao SQ, Lee K, Huang XS, Yang WY, et al. AUNX1, a novel locus responsible for X linked recessive auditory and peripheral neuropathy, maps to Xq23-27.3. Journal of Medical Genetics. 2006;**43**(7):e33

[112] Starr A, Sininger YS, Pratt H. The varieties of auditory neuropathy. Journal of Basic and Clinical Physiology and Pharmacology. 2000;**11**(3):215-230

[113] Rogers R, Kimberling WJ, Starr A, Kirschhofer K, Cohn E, Kenyon J, et al. The genetics of auditory neuropathy. Auditory Neuropathy: A New Perspective on Hearing Disorders San Diego: Singular Publishing Co. 2001:165-182

[114] Almishaal AA, Saleh S, Alferaih H, Alhelo O. Prevalence, risk factors, and audiological characteristics of auditory neuropathy. International Journal of Audiology. 2021;1-9

[115] Shapiro SM, Nakamura H. Bilirubin and the auditory system. Journal of Perinatology: Official Journal of the California Perinatal Association. 2001;**21**(Suppl. 1):S52-S55; discussion S59-62

[116] Agrawal Y, Platz EA, Niparko JK. Prevalence of hearing loss and differences by demographic characteristics among US adults: Data from the National Health and Nutrition Examination Survey, 1999-2004. Archives of Internal Medicine. 2008;**168**(14):1522-1530

[117] Bowl MR, Dawson SJ. Age-related hearing loss. Cold Spring Harbor Perspectives in Medicine. 2019;**9**(8):a033217

[118] Christensen K, Frederiksen H, Hoffman HJ. Genetic and environmental influences on self-reported reduced hearing in the old and oldest old. Journal of the American Geriatrics Society. 2001;**49**(11):1512-1517

[119] Schuknecht HF, Gacek MR. Cochlear pathology in presbycusis. The Annals of Otology, Rhinology, and Laryngology. 1993;**102**(suppl. 1):1-16

[120] Schuknecht HF. Presbycusis. Transactions of the American Laryngological, Rhinological and Otological Society, Inc. 1955;**65**(6): 402-419

[121] Wingfield A, Panizzon M, Grant MD, Toomey R, Kremen WS, Franz CE, et al. A twin-study of genetic contributions to hearing acuity in late middle age. The Journals of Gerontology: Series A. 2007;**62**(11):1294-1299

[122] Gates GA, Couropmitree NN, Myers RH. Genetic associations in age-related hearing thresholds. Archives of Otolaryngology—Head & Neck, Surgery. 1999;**125**(6):654-659

[123] Boucher S, Tai FWJ, Delmaghani S, Lelli A, Singh-Estivalet A, Dupont T, et al. Ultrarare heterozygous pathogenic variants of genes causing dominant forms of early-onset deafness underlie severe presbycusis. Proceedings of the National Academy of Sciences of the United States of America. 2020;**117**(49):31278-31289

[124] Payne JA, Xu J-C, Haas M, Lytle CY, Ward D, Forbush BJ. Primary structure, functional expression, and chromosomal localization of the bumetanide-sensitive Na-K-Cl cotransporter in human colon. Journal of Biological Chemistry. 1995;**270**(30):17977-17985

[125] Crouch JJ, Sakaguchi N, Lytle C, Schulte BA. Immunohistochemical localization of the Na-K-Cl co-transporter (NKCC1) in the gerbil inner ear. Journal of Histochemistry & Cytochemistry. 1997;**45**(6):773-778

[126] Schulte BA, Steel KP. Expression of α and β subunit isoforms of Na, K-ATPase in the mouse inner ear and changes with mutations at the Wv or Sld loci. Hearing Research. 1994;**78**(1):65-76

[127] Xia A-P, Kikuchi T, Hozawa K, Katori Y, Takasaka TJ. Expression of connexin 26 and Na, K-ATPase in the developing mouse cochlear lateral wall: Functional implications. Brain Research. 1999;**846**(1):106-111

[128] Salt A, Demott JJI, Physiology IE. Pathophysiology. London WP: Physical processes underlying homeostasis of cochlear endolymph; 1999

[129] Diaz RC, Vazquez AE, Dou H, Wei D, Cardell EL, Lingrel J, et al. Conservation of hearing by simultaneous mutation of Na, K-ATPase and NKCC1. Journal of the Association for Research in Otolaryngology: JARO. 2007;**8**(4):422-434

[130] Kharkovets T, Hardelin J-P, Safieddine S, Schweizer M, El-Amraoui A, Petit C, et al. KCNQ4, a K+ channel mutated in a form of dominant deafness, is expressed in the inner ear and the central auditory pathway. Proceedings of the National Academy of Sciences of the United States of America. 2000;**97**(8):4333-4338

[131] Marres H, van Ewijk M, Huygen P, Kunst H, van Camp G, Coucke P, et al. Inherited nonsyndromic hearing loss: An audiovestibular study in a large family with autosomal dominant progressive hearing loss related to DFNA2. Archives of Otolaryngology—Head & Neck Surgery. 1997;**123**(6):573-577

[132] Kubisch C, Schroeder BC, Friedrich T, Lütjohann B, El-Amraoui A, Marlin S, et al. KCNQ4, a novel potassium channel expressed in sensory outer hair cells, is mutated in dominant deafness. Cell. 1999;**96**(3):437-446

[133] Coucke P, Van Camp G, Djoyodiharjo B, Smith SD, Frants RR, Padberg GW, et al. Linkage of autosomal dominant hearing loss to the short arm of chromosome 1 in two families. New England Journal of Medicine. 1994;**331**(7):425-431

[134] Kamada F, Kure S, Kudo T, Suzuki Y, Oshima T, Ichinohe A, et al. A novel KCNQ4 one-base deletion

in a large pedigree with hearing loss: Implication for the genotype–phenotype correlation. Journal of Human Genetics. 2006;**51**(5):455-460

[135] Van Eyken E, Van Laer L, Fransen E, Topsakal V, Lemkens N, Laureys W, et al. KCNQ4: A gene for age-related hearing impairment? Human Mutation. 2006;**27**(10):1007-1016

[136] Osman AA, Saito M, Makepeace C, Permutt MA, Schlesinger P, Mueckler MJ. Wolframin expression induces novel ion channel activity in endoplasmic reticulum membranes and increases intracellular calcium. Journal of Biological Chemistry. 2003;**278**(52):52755-52762

[137] Wolfram D. Diabetes mellitus and simple optic atrophy among siblings. Mayo Clinic Proceedings. 1938;**1938**:715-718

[138] Bespalova IN, Van Camp G, Bom JS, Brown DJ, Cryns K, AT DW, et al. Mutations in the Wolfram syndrome 1 gene (WFS1) are a common cause of low frequency sensorineural hearing loss. Human Molecular Genetics. 2001;**10**(22):2501-2508

[139] Van Camp G, Kunst H, Flothmann K, McGuirt W, Wauters J, Marres H, et al. A gene for autosomal dominant hearing impairment (DFNA14) maps to a region on chromosome 4p16. 3 that does not overlap the DFNA6 locus. Journal of Medical Genetics. 1999;**36**(7):532-536

[140] Lesperance MM, Hail JW III, Bess FH, Fukushima K, Jain PK, Plopils B, et al. A gene for autosomal dominant nonsyndromic hereditary hearing impairment maps to 4p16.3. Human Molecular Genetics. 1995;**4**(10):1967-1972

[141] Kytövuori L, Hannula S, Mäki-Torkko E, Sorri M, Majamaa KJHR. A nonsynonymous mutation in the WFS1 gene in a Finnish family with age-related hearing impairment. Hearing Research. 2017;**355**:97-101

[142] Pineda M, Fernández E, Torrents D, Estévez R, López C, Camps M, et al. Identification of a membrane protein, LAT-2, that co-expresses with 4F2 heavy chain, an L-type amino acid transport activity with broad specificity for small and large zwitterionic amino acids. Journal of Biological Chemistry. 1999;**274**(28):19738-19744

[143] Uetsuka S, Ogata G, Nagamori S, Isozumi N, Nin F, Yoshida T, et al. Molecular architecture of the stria vascularis membrane transport system, which is essential for physiological functions of the mammalian cochlea. European Journal of Neuroscience. 2015;**42**(3):1984-2002

[144] Guarch ME, Font-Llitjós M, Murillo-Cuesta S, Errasti-Murugarren E, Celaya AM, Girotto G, et al. Mutations in L-type amino acid transporter-2 support SLC7A8 as a novel gene involved in age-related hearing loss. eLife. 2018;**7**:e31511

[145] Wallace DC. Mitochondrial DNA in aging and disease. Scientific American. 1997;**277**(2):40-47

[146] Fischel-Ghodsian N, Bykhovskaya Y, Taylor K, Kahen T, Cantor R, Ehrenman K, et al. Temporal bone analysis of patients with presbycusis reveals high frequency of mitochondrial mutations. Hearing Research. 1997;**110**(1-2):147-154

[147] Bai U, Seidman MD, Hinojosa R, Quirk WS. Mitochondrial DNA deletions associated with aging and possibly presbycusis: A human archival temporal bone study. American Journal of Otology. 1997;**18**(4):449-453

[148] Seidman MD, Bai U, Khan MJ, Quirk WS. Mitochondrial DNA deletions

associated with aging and presbyacusis. American Journal of Otology. 1997;**123**(10):1039-1045

[149] Markaryan A, Nelson EG, Hinojosa RJ. Major arc mitochondrial DNA deletions in cytochrome c oxidase-deficient human cochlear spiral ganglion cells. Acta Oto-laryngologica. 2010;**130**(7):780-787

[150] Lu J, Holmgren AJ. The thioredoxin antioxidant system. Free Radical Biology & Medicine. 2014;**66**:75-87

[151] Ying WJ. NAD+/NADH and NADP+/NADPH in cellular functions and cell death: Regulation and biological consequences. Antioxidants & Redox Signaling. 2008;**10**(2):179-206

[152] Tadros SF, D'Souza M, Zhu X, Frisina RD. Gene expression changes for antioxidants pathways in the mouse cochlea: Relations to age-related hearing deficits. PLOS ONE. 2014;**9**(2):e90279

[153] Aburto MR, Magariños M, Leon Y, Varela-Nieto I, Sanchez-Calderon HJ. AKT signaling mediates IGF-I survival actions on otic neural progenitors. PLOS ONE. 2012;**7**(1):e30790

[154] Tafra R, Brakus SM, Vukojevic K, Kablar B, Colovic Z, Saraga-Babic M. Interplay of proliferation and proapoptotic and antiapoptotic factors is revealed in the early human inner ear development. Otology & Neurotology: Official Publication of the American Otological Society, American Neurotology Society [and] European Academy of Otology and Neurotology. 2014;**35**(4):695-703

[155] Rodríguez-de la Rosa L, Sánchez-Calderón H, Contreras J, Murillo-Cuesta S, Falagan S, Avendano C, et al. Comparative gene expression study of the vestibular organ of the Igf1 deficient mouse using whole-transcript arrays. Hearing Research. 2015;**330**:62-77

[156] Degerman E, Rauch U, Lindberg S, Caye-Thomasen P, Hultgårdh A, Magnusson M. Expression of insulin signalling components in the sensory epithelium of the human saccule. Cell and Tissue Research. 2013;**352**(3):469-478

[157] Riva C, Donadieu E, Magnan J, Lavieille J-PJ. Age-related hearing loss in CD/1 mice is associated to ROS formation and HIF target proteins up-regulation in the cochlea. Experimental Gerontology. 2007;**42**(4):327-336

[158] Attias J, Zarchi O, Nageris BI, Laron Z. Cochlear hearing loss in patients with Laron syndrome. European Archives of Oto-rhino-laryngology: Official Journal of the European Federation of Oto-Rhino-Laryngological Societies (EUFOS): Affiliated with the German Society for Oto-Rhino-Laryngology—Head and Neck Surgery. 2012;**269**(2):461-466

[159] Prado-Barreto VM, Salvatori R, Santos Junior RC, Brandão-Martins MB, Correa EA, Garcez FB, et al. Hearing status in adult individuals with lifetime, untreated isolated growth hormone deficiency. Otolaryngology—Head and Neck Surgery: Official Journal of American Academy of Otolaryngology-Head and Neck Surgery. 2014;**150**(3):464-471

[160] Ester WA, van Duyvenvoorde HA, de Wit CC, Broekman AJ, Ruivenkamp CA, Govaerts LC, et al. Two short children born small for gestational age with insulin-like growth factor 1 receptor haploinsufficiency illustrate the heterogeneity of its phenotype. Journal of Clinical Endocrinology and Metabolism. 2009;**94**(12):4717-4727

[161] Hermans-Borgmeyer I, SuÈsens U, Borgmeyer U. Developmental expression of the estrogen receptor-related receptor γ in the nervous system during

mouse embryogenesis. Mechanisms of Development. 2000;**97**(1-2):197-199

[162] Hultcrantz M, Simonoska R, Stenberg AE. Estrogen and hearing: a summary of recent investigations. Acta Oto-laryngologica. 2006;**126**(1):10-14

[163] McCullar JS, ECJ O. Cellular targets of estrogen signaling in regeneration of inner ear sensory epithelia. Hearing Research. 2009;**252**(1-2):61-70

[164] Helzner EP, Cauley JA, Pratt SR, Wisniewski SR, Zmuda JM, Talbott EO, et al. Race and sex differences in age-related hearing loss: The Health, Aging and Body Composition Study. Journal of the American Geriatrics Society. 2005;**53**(12):2119-2127

[165] Pearson JD, Morrell CH, Gordon-Salant S, Brant LJ, Metter EJ, Klein LL, et al. Gender differences in a longitudinal study of age-associated hearing loss. Journal of the Acoustical Society of America. 1995;**97**(2):1196-1205

[166] Nolan LS, Maier H, Hermans-Borgmeyer I, Girotto G, Ecob R, Pirastu N, et al. Estrogen-related receptor gamma and hearing function: Evidence of a role in humans and mice. Neurobiology of Aging. 2013;**34**(8):2077.e2071-2077.e2079

[167] Manche SK, Jangala M, Dudekula D, Koralla M, Akka JJ. Polymorphisms in folate metabolism genes are associated with susceptibility to presbycusis. Life Sciences. 2018;**196**:77-83

[168] Friedman RA, Van Laer L, Huentelman MJ, Sheth SS, Van Eyken E, Corneveaux JJ, et al. GRM7 variants confer susceptibility to age-related hearing impairment. Human Molecular Genetics. 2009;**18**(4):785-796

[169] Newman DL, Fisher LM, Ohmen J, Parody R, Fong C-T, Frisina ST, et al. GRM7 variants associated with age-related hearing loss based on auditory perception. Hearing Research. 2012;**294**(1-2):125, 132

[170] Van Laer L, Huyghe JR, Hannula S, Van Eyken E, Stephan DA, Mäki-Torkko E, et al. A genome-wide association study for age-related hearing impairment in the Saami. European Journal of Human Genetics. 2010;**18**(6):685-693

[171] Han Y, Mu Y, Li X, Xu P, Tong J, Liu Z, et al. Grhl2 deficiency impairs otic development and hearing ability in a zebrafish model of the progressive dominant hearing loss DFNA28. Human Molecular Genetics. 2011;**20**(16):3213-3226

[172] Peters LM, Anderson DW, Griffith AJ, Grundfast KM, San Agustin TB, Madeo AC, et al. Mutation of a transcription factor, TFCP2L3, causes progressive autosomal dominant hearing loss, DFNA28. Human Molecular Genetics. 2002;**11**(23):2877-2885

[173] Vona B, Nanda I, Neuner C, Müller T, Haaf TJ. Confirmation of GRHL2 as the gene for the DFNA28 locus. American Journal of Medical Genetics. Part A. 2013;**161**(8):2060-2065

[174] Van Laer L, Van Eyken E, Fransen E, Huyghe JR, Topsakal V, Hendrickx J-J, et al. The grainyhead like 2 gene (GRHL2), alias TFCP2L3, is associated with age-related hearing impairment. Human Molecular Genetics. 2008;**17**(2):159-169

[175] Herzog B, Pellet-Many C, Britton G, Hartzoulakis B, Zachary IC. VEGF binding to NRP1 is essential for VEGF stimulation of endothelial cell migration, complex formation between NRP1 and VEGFR2, and signaling via FAK Tyr407 phosphorylation. Molecular Biology of the Cell. 2011;**22**(15):2766-2776

[176] Coate TM, Spita NA, Zhang KD, Isgrig KT, Kelley MW. Neuropilin-2/Semaphorin-3F-mediated repulsion promotes inner hair cell innervation by spiral ganglion neurons. ELife. 2015;**4**:e07830

[177] Salehi P, Ge MX, Gundimeda U, Michelle Baum L, Lael Cantu H, Lavinsky J, et al. Role of Neuropilin-1/Semaphorin-3A signaling in the functional and morphological integrity of the cochlea. PLoS Genetics. 2017;**13**(10):e1007048

[178] Di Palma F, Pellegrino R, Noben-Trauth KJ. Genomic structure, alternative splice forms and normal and mutant alleles of cadherin 23 (Cdh23). Gene. 2001;**281**(1-2):31-41

[179] Hwang J-H, Chen J-C, Hsu C-J, Yang W-S, Liu T-C. Plasma reactive oxygen species levels are correlated with severity of age-related hearing impairment in humans. Neurobiology of Aging. 2012;**33**(9):1920-1926

[180] Bouzid A, Smeti I, Chakroun A, Loukil S, Gibriel AA, Grati M, et al. CDH23 methylation status and presbycusis risk in elderly women. Frontiers in Aging Neuroscience. 2018;**10**:1-7

[181] Baguley D, McFerran D, Hall DJ. Tinnitus. Lancet. 2013;**382**(9904):1600-1607

[182] Eladawy II, Abou Elhassan H. Prevalence of tinnitus among the attendees of the audio-vestibular unit at Al-Zahraa University Hospital, Cairo, Egypt. International Journal of Medical Arts. 2015;**13**(3):2

[183] Khedr EM, Ahmed MA, Shawky OA, Mohamed ES, El Attar GS, Mohammad KA. Epidemiological study of chronic tinnitus in Assiut, Egypt. Neuroepidemiology. 2010;**35**(1):45-52

[184] Michikawa T, Nishiwaki Y, Kikuchi Y, Saito H, Mizutari K, Okamoto M, et al. Prevalence and factors associated with tinnitus: A community-based study of Japanese elders. Journal of Epidemiology. 2010;**20**:271-276

[185] Fujii K, Nagata C, Nakamura K, Kawachi T, Takatsuka N, Oba S, et al. Prevalence of tinnitus in community-dwelling Japanese adults. Journal of Epidemiology. 2011;**21**(4):299-304

[186] Kojima T, Kanzaki S, Oishi N, Ogawa KJ. Clinical characteristics of patients with tinnitus evaluated with the Tinnitus Sample Case History Questionnaire in Japan: A case series. PLOS ONE. 2017;**12**(8):e0180609

[187] Lasisi AO, Abiona T, Gureje O. Tinnitus in the elderly: Profile, correlates, and impact in the Nigerian Study of Ageing. Otolaryngology—Head and Neck Surgery: Official Journal of American Academy of Otolaryngology-Head and Neck Surgery. 2010;**143**(4):510-515

[188] Sogebi OA. Characterization of tinnitus in Nigeria. Auris Nasus Larynx. 2013;**40**(4):356-360

[189] Biswas R, Lugo A, Akeroyd MA, Schlee W, Gallus S, Hall D. Tinnitus prevalence in Europe: A multi-country cross-sectional population study. The Lancet Regional Health—Europe. 2022;**12**:100250

[190] Choi JS, Yu AJ, Voelker CC, Doherty JK, Oghalai JS, Fisher LM. Prevalence of tinnitus and associated factors among Asian Americans: Results from a national sample. Laryngoscope. 2020;**130**(12):E933-E940

[191] Bhatt JM, Lin HW, Bhattacharyya N. Prevalence, severity, exposures, and treatment patterns of tinnitus in the United States. JAMA

Otolaryngology—Head & Neck Surgery. 2016;**142**(10):959-965

[192] Mahboubi H, Oliaei S, Kiumehr S, Dwabe S, Djalilian HR. The prevalence and characteristics of tinnitus in the youth population of the United States. Otology/Neurotology. 2013;**123**(8):2001-2008

[193] Sindhusake D, Golding M, Newall P, Rubin G, Jakobsen K, Mitchell PJ. Risk factors for tinnitus in a population of older adults: the blue mountains hearing study. Ear and Hearing. 2003;**24**(6):501-507

[194] Kvestad E, Czajkowski N, Engdahl B, Hoffman HJ, Tambs K. Low heritability of tinnitus: Results from the second Nord-Trøndelag health study. Archives of Otorhinolaryngology-Head & Neck Surgery. 2010;**136**(2):178-182

[195] Vona B, Nanda I, Shehata-Dieler W, Haaf T. Genetics of tinnitus: Still in its infancy. Frontiers in Neuroscience. 2017;**11**:236

Chapter 7

Nonreceptor Protein Kinases and Phosphatases Necessary for Auditory Function

Sadaf Naz

Abstract

Phosphorylation is one of the most common posttranslational protein modifications. It has multiple roles in cell signaling during development as well as for maintenance of diverse functions of an organism. Protein kinases and phosphatases control phosphorylation and play critical roles in cellular processes from cell birth to cell death. Discovery of hearing-loss-associated gene variants in humans and the study of animal models have identified a crucial role of a plethora of protein phosphatases and kinases in the inner ear. In this review, those nonreceptor kinases or phosphatases are discussed, which are encoded by genes implicated in causing inherited hearing loss in humans or in mouse mutants. These studies have served to highlight the essential roles of protein kinases and phosphatases pathways to the function of the auditory system. However, the inner-ear-specific substrates for most of these enzymes remain to be discovered, as do the mechanisms of disease due to the variants in the genes that encode these proteins.

Keywords: audition, deafness, dephosphorylation, hearing, phosphorylation

1. Introduction

Different protein posttranslational modifications have been identified, which are necessary for hearing [1]. Among these, protein phosphorylation is a prominent and an important contributor to the development of the ear and control of audition. Phosphorylation is carried out by kinases using γ-phosphate from adenosine triphosphate as a donor to any of the three hydroxylated amino acids within the target protein. The removal of the phosphate group from the phosphorylated tyrosine, serine, or threonine residues of the proteins is catalyzed by phosphatases. Phosphorylation and dephosphorylation serve to change the polarity of the target proteins with profound consequences for protein conformation and interaction with other proteins [2].

Enzymes controlling phosphorylation can be categorized into receptor or nonreceptor protein kinases and phosphatases. Many phosphorylated proteins as well as enzymes that control these reactions have important roles in the auditory system [1]. Though variants in all genes encoding these proteins do not result in deafness; variants of some protein kinases and phosphatases have been reported to cause genetic hearing loss in humans or mice models, and these are presented here. Receptor kinases or receptor phosphatases important for hearing are discussed elsewhere [3] and are excluded from the discussion, as are those kinases or phosphatases that catalyze the phosphorylation or dephosphorylation of non-proteinaceous biomolecules.

Variants of most of the genes encoding protein kinases or phosphatases have been reported to cause syndromic hearing loss (**Table 1**). In syndromic cases, deafness is just one of the accompanying features in a spectrum of other disorder/s affecting different organs. Syndromic deafness occurs due to the importance of the protein to other systems besides the ear. The hearing loss may be present in all individuals affected by a particular syndrome, while for others it affects only a few patients diagnosed with that syndrome. In contrast, hearing loss is the sole manifestation in an individual with nonsyndromic deafness [4].

1.1 Auditory system and hearing

The auditory system in humans has distinct parts, which include the outer ear, the middle ear, and the inner ear. Sound is perceived and processed by the ear with the final stimulus conveyed to the auditory cortex in the brain. The outer and the middle ears play important roles in conveying the sound to the cochlea within the inner ear. The cochlea is a coiled structure and contains the organ of Corti, which has the sensory receptors, termed as outer and inner hair cells. All hair cells have mechanosensitive microvilli projections at their apical ends, termed as stereocilia, which have important roles for their function [3]. True cilia, called the kinocilia, are also present, but these disappear early during maturation of the mammalian auditory system. The hair cells amplify the sound and transduce it into an electrical stimulus. The electric stimulus from the inner hair cells is finally conveyed to the brain via the spiral ganglion neurons.

1.2 Hearing loss and its types

A partial or a complete inability to hear sound is a common sensory disorder and is termed as hearing loss or deafness. Worldwide, both children and adults are affected, and approximately 430 million individuals are reported to suffer from a hearing loss (World Health Organization, 2021, https://www.who.int/news-room/fact-sheets/detail/deafness-and-hearing-loss). Deafness is categorized into four types on the basis of the affected part. Conductive hearing loss arises as a result of impedance of passage of sound through the external ear and/or the middle ear. Sensorineural hearing loss is caused by malfunction of the inner ear (cochlea or auditory nerve). Mixed hearing loss is a combination of both conductive and sensorineural hearing loss. Central auditory processing disorder results due to damage or malfunction at the cranial nerves, the cerebral cortex, or the auditory brain stem [4].

On the basis of onset, hearing loss can be prelingual or postlingual. Prelingual hearing loss occurs during infancy, before the development of speech. Postlingual hearing loss appears after normal speech development; either during childhood or adulthood. Hearing of an individual is measured in decibels (dB HL). A normal hearing threshold is 15 dB HL while a disabling hearing loss is defined as a threshold of 35 db HL or above for the better hearing ear. Hearing loss is divided into five types on the basis of severity [4]: mild hearing loss (hearing threshold 26–40 dB HL), moderate hearing loss (hearing threshold 41–55 dB), moderately severe hearing loss (hearing threshold 56–70 dB), severe hearing loss (hearing threshold 71–90 dB), and profound hearing loss (hearing threshold >90 dB). The extent of hearing loss may be stable throughout a person's life, or it may progress and worsen over time. Genetic hearing loss contributes to at least

Name	HGNC/OMIM	Alias	Function	Human Disorder/OMIM/Inheritance/ OR mouse phenotype	Reference*
Protein Kinases					
Dual-Specificity Kinases (CMGC group)					
Dual-specificity tYrosine phosphorylation-Regulated Kinase 1A	DYRK1A/ 600,855	DYRK1	General role in the MAPK pathway	Mental retardation, autosomal dominant 7/614104/AD	[11]
Dual-Specificity Kinases (STE Group)					
Mitogen-Activated Protein Kinase kinase 1	MAP2K1/615279	PRKMK1 MAPKK1 MKK1 MEK1	General role in MAPK phosphorylation	Noonan syndrome-like/NA/AD Cardiofaciocutaneous syndrome 3/615279/ AD	[12] [13]
Protein Serine/Threonine Kinases (AGC Group)					
CDC42-Binding Protein kinase, Beta	CDC42BPB/614062	MRCKB	General role in proliferation	Neurodevelopmental phenotype/NA/AD	[15]
Protein Kinase C, Beta	PRKCB/176970	PRKCB1 PKCB	Histone H3 phosphorylation	Meniere's disease with hearing loss/NA/AD	[23]
PRotein Kinase C, Gamma	PRKCG/176980	PKCC PKCG	General role in development	Spinocerebellar Ataxia 14/605361/AD	[20]
Protein Serine/Threonine Kinases (AGC CAMK Group)					
Ribosomal Protein S6 Kinase A3	RPS6KA3/300075	ISPK1 MAPKAPK1B RSK2	Histone H3 and PDZ domain-containing proteins' phosphorylation	Coffin-Lowry Syndrome/303600/XLD	[21]
Protein Serine/Threonine Kinases (CAMK Group)					
Calcium/Calmodulin-dependent Serine Protein Kinase	CASK/300172	CMG LIN2	Interacts with prestin and whirlin in the inner ear	Intellectual developmental disorder with microcephaly and pontine and cerebellar hypoplasia/300749/ XLD	[7]
Mitogen-Activated Protein Kinase-Activated Protein Kinase 5	MAPKAPK5/ 606,723	MK5 PRAK	Heat shock protein HSP27 phosphorylation	Developmental disorder with hearing loss/ NA/AR	[22]

Name	HGNC/OMIM	Alias	Function	Human Disorder/OMIM/Inheritance/ OR mouse phenotype	Reference*
Serine/Threonine protein Kinase 11	STK11/	LKB1	Maintenance of stereocilia by phosphorylation of radixin, eosin and moesin, Planar cell polarity, formation of cochlear hair cells	No hearing loss phenotype in humans/Ear specific, *Atoh1*^{cre}, *Lkb1*$^{-/-}$ mice have hearing deficits	[32]
Protein Serine/Threonine Kinases (CMGC Group)					
Cyclin-Dependent Kinase 5	CDK5/123831	PSSALRE	Maintenance of stereocilia by phosphorylation of radixin, eosin and moesin	No hearing loss phenotype in humans/ Ear specific, *Atoh1*$^{Cre/+}$;*Cdk5*$^{lox/lox}$ mice have hearing loss	[10]
Cyclin-Dependent Kinase 8	CDK8/603184	K35	Component of RNA polymerase II holoenzyme where kinase function phosphorylates POLR2A	Intellectual developmental disorder with hypotonia and behavioral abnormalities/ 618,748/AD	[16]
Cyclin-Dependent Kinase 9	CDK9/ 603,251	CTK1 PITALRE	Phosphorylates POLR2A	CHARGE syndrome-like/NA/AR	[17]
Cyclin-Dependent Kinase 10	CDK10/603464	PISSLRE	General role in ciliogenesis and elongation of the primary cilium	Al Kaissi Syndrome/617694/AR	[18]
Cyclin-Dependent Kinase 13	CDK13/ 603,309	CDC2L5 CHED	Phosphorylates the large subunit RBP1	Wolfram-like syndrome/NA/AR	[19]
Mitogen-Activated Protein Kinase 1	MAPK1/176948	ERK2, p42MAPK PRKM1 PRKM2	Survival of hair cells in response to noise and multiple general roles in MAPK signaling	No hearing loss phenotype in humans/ Ear-specific knockout mice are susceptible to noise-induced hearing loss	[33]
Protein Serine/Threonine kinases (STE Group)					
Mitogen-Activated Protein Kinase Kinase Kinase 1	MAP3K1/600982	MAPKKK1 MEK MEKK1	Phosphorylation of MAPK14 in cochlea and general role in MAPK signaling	No hearing loss phenotype in humans/ Knockout mice are deaf	[28, 29]

Name	HGNC/OMIM	Alias	Function	Human Disorder/OMIM/Inheritance/ OR mouse phenotype	Reference*
Mitogen-Activated Protein Kinase Kinase Kinase 4	MAP3K4/602425	MAPKKK4 MEKK4 MTK1	FGFR1 signaling control and general role in MAPK signaling	No hearing loss phenotype in humans/ Knock-in *Mekk4*$^{K1361R/K1361R/}$ mice are deaf	[30]
Mitogen-Activated Protein Kinase Kinase Kinase 7	MAP3K7/602614	TAK1a TAK1b TAK1c TAK1d	Phosphorylation of MAPK14, mediates BMP and TGFB signaling, general role in MAPK signaling	Cardiospondylocarpofacial syndrome/157800/AD Frontometaphyseal dysplasia 2/617137/AD	[14]
Myosin IIIA	MYO3A/606808	NA	Self-regulation of MYO3A motor domain activity	Deafness, autosomal recessive 30/607101/ AR Deafness, autosomal dominant/NA/AD	[5] [36]
p21 Protein-Activated Kinase 1	PAK1/602590	NA	Maintenance of hair cells and stereocilia by phosphorylation of cofilin and ezrin-radixin-moesin (ERM) and βII-spectrin	No hearing loss phenotype in humans/ Knockout mice have hearing loss	[31]
Protein Serine/Threonine Kinases (TKL Group)					
B-RAF protooncogene, serine/ threonine kinase	BRAF/ 164,757	BRAF1 RAFB1	MAPK/ERK pathway	LEOPARD syndrome 3,613,707/AD	[24]
Mitogen-Activated Protein Kinase Kinase Kinase 20	MAP3K20/609479	MLTK MRK ZAK	MAPK/ERK Pathway, general role in MAPK signaling	Split-foot malformation with mesoaxial polydactyly/ 616,890/AR	[26]
RAF1 protooncogene, serine/ threonine kinase	RAF1/164760	CRAF	RAS/MAPK pathway	Leopard syndrome 2/ 611,554/AD	[25]
Protein Tyrosine Kinases, non-receptor class (TK Group)					
ABL protooncogene 1, nonreceptor Tyrosine Kinase	ABL1/189980	ABL	General role in cell cycle function	Congenital heart defects and skeletal malformations syndrome/ 617,602/AD	[40, 41]

Name	HGNC/OMIM	Alias	Function	Human Disorder/OMIM/Inheritance/ OR mouse phenotype	Reference*
Bruton Agammaglobulinemia Tyrosine Kinase	BTK/300300	ATK BPK	General role in maturation of B cells. Antibody response is thought to reduce hearing loss occurring due to infections	Agammaglobulinemia, X-linked 1/300755/ XLR	[42]
Protein Phosphatases					
Atypical Protein Phosphatases (HAD fold, EYA Family)					
EYA transcriptional coactivator and phosphatase 1	EYA1/601653	NA	Development of components of the outer middle and inner ear	Branchiootorenal syndrome 1, with or without cataracts/ 113,650/AD Branchiootic Syndrome 1/ 602,588/AD	[46] [47]
EYA transcriptional coactivator and phosphatase 4	EYA4/603550	NA	Post-developmental function of Organ of corti	Deafness, autosomal dominant 10/ 601,316/AD Cardiomyopathy, dilated, 1 J/ 605,362/AD	[49] [50]
Dual-Specificity Phosphatases (CC1 fold, DSP family)					
Cell Division Cycle 14A	CDC14A/603504	CDC14	Conservation of hair cells	Deafness, autosomal recessive 32, with or without immotile sperm/608653/AR	[52, 53]
Dual-Specificity Phosphatase 1	DUSP1/600714	CL100 PTPN10 MKP1	MAPK dephosphorylation, Regulation of oxidative balance and inflammatory immune response in the ear	No hearing loss phenotype in humans/ Knockout mice have a progressive hearing loss	[55, 56]
Dual-Specificity Phosphatase 6	DUSP6/602748	MKP3 PYST1	MAPK1 dephosphorylation, Negative regulation of FGF signaling pathway in ear development	Hypogonadotropic hypogonadism 19 with or without anosmia/615269/ AD (HL in some patients)	[59]
Dual-Specificity Phosphatases (CC1 fold, PTEN family)					
Phosphatase and Tensin Homolog	PTEN/601728	MMAC1 PTEN1	Cell cycle regulation and exit of auditory sensory progenitors	Cowden syndrome 1/ 158,350/AD	[64]

DOI: http://dx.doi.org/10.5772/intechopen.105425

Name	HGNC/OMIM	Alias	Function	Human Disorder/OMIM/Inheritance/ OR mouse phenotype	Reference*
Protein Tyrosine Phosphatases, nonreceptor-type (CC1 fold, PTP family)					
Protein-Tyrosine Phosphatase, nonreceptor-type, 11	PTPN11/176876	PTP2C SHP2	Regulates RAS/MAPK signaling pathway	Leopard Syndrome 1/ 151,100/AD Nonsyndromic hearing loss/NA/AD Noonan Syndrome 1/ 163,950/AD	[65] [68] [66]

*HGNC=HUGO Gene Nomenclature Committee, OMIM = Online Mendelian Inheritance in Man, AD = Autosomal Dominant, AR = Autosomal Recessive, XLD = X-linked Dominant, XLR = X-linked Recessive, CMGC=Cyclin-dependent kinases (CDK), Mitogen-activated protein kinases (MAPK), Glycogen synthase kinase (GSK3) and CDC-like kinase (CLK) group of protein kinases, STE = Sterile group of Kinases, CAMK=Ca^{2+}/calModulin-dependent protein Kinase, TKL = Tyrosine Kinase Like, TK = Tyrosine Kinase, AGC = cyclic AMP-dependent kinases (PKA), cGMP-dependent kinases, and the diacylglycerol-activated/phospholipid-dependent kinase PKC group of kinases, HAD = Haloacid Dehalogenase, EYA = Eyes Absent, CC1 = Cysteine-based Class 1, DSP=Dual-specific phosphatase, PTP=Protein Tyrosine Phosphatase, NA = Not available.*Reference to the report of auditory phenotype in mice is only provided if hearing loss has not been described in humans. Classification of the protein kinases and the protein phosphatases is from Manning et al. 2002 [ref. 6] and Chen et al. 2018 [ref. 43], respectively.*

Table 1.
Nonreceptor protein kinases and phosphatases implicated in hearing loss.

50% of all deafness cases, while the remaining is attributed to environmental factors such as exposure to loud noise, infections, or ototoxic drugs [4].

1.3 Genes in hearing and deafness

Genetic deafness can be monogenic in affected individuals or may have a more complex etiology. Many proteins orchestrate human hearing, and variants in hundreds of genes have been implicated in causing deafness. Some of these genes encode structural components within the auditory system; others encode proteins necessary for the function of the ear. Variants of many genes have been reported to cause structural defects of the ear with or without hearing loss in humans [4].

Inherited hearing loss has different modes of inheritance in different families [4]. These include autosomal dominant, autosomal recessive, X-linked, or mitochondrial inheritance. The autosomal forms are more commonly encountered as compared with the other types of inheritance patterns. Most of the dominantly inherited gene variants in humans cause postlingual, progressive, moderate to severe sensorineural hearing loss. In contrast, the majority of recessively inherited variants result in prelingual severe to profound sensorineural deafness [4]. However, exceptions exist for both dominant and recessive inherited hearing loss cases in which the phenotypic pattern for recessive forms resembles that of the dominant disorders or vice versa [5].

2. Protein kinases

Hundreds of protein kinases are encoded in the human genome and constitute more than 2.5% of the coding genes [6]. These enzymes phosphorylate the hydroxyl groups of the target proteins at the serine/threonine residues (protein serine/threonine kinases) or act on the tyrosine residues (protein tyrosine kinases) or both (dual-specificity kinases). Generally, nonreceptor kinases are intracellular cytoplasmic or nuclear proteins. Variants of most of these genes cause hearing loss in only a subset of the affected individuals, suggesting a degree of redundancy for the function of the auditory system. One such gene is *CASK*; patients with *CASK* variants have an Intellectual developmental disorder with microcephaly and pontine and cerebellar hypoplasia syndrome, and only a few individuals also have a hearing loss [7]. Interestingly, CASK has been shown to interact with whirlin and prestin in the inner ear; [8, 9] two proteins that are vital to hearing.

Sometimes, hearing loss phenotype is not investigated or observed in mouse models for many of the genes, which are known to cause deafness in humans. In other cases, targeted disruption of a gene, for example, *Cdk5*, causes lethality in mice, necessitating the development of animal models with selective deletion of the gene of interest in the inner ear [10] in order to determine the effect of the absence of the protein in the auditory system. Multiple studies on mouse models with deafness have suggested that some of the kinases important for hearing have roles in the kinocilia formation or maintenance of the stereocilia [9].

2.1 Dual-specificity kinases

DYRK1A is a dual-specificity kinase, which has been implicated in individuals with mental retardation and outer ear morphological defects (**Table 1**). Some individuals also experience hearing loss due to *DYRK1A* variants [11]. DYRK1A autophosphorylates itself at both serine/threonine and tyrosine residues, and thus controls its own activity. Another dual-specificity kinase, MAP2K1 is required for activation of MAPK by phosphorylating both serine and tyrosine residues. Variants of *MAP2K1* have been associated with hearing loss in a few patients diagnosed with either of two different human syndromes (**Table 1**), as an accompanying feature to the cardiovascular defects [12, 13].

2.2 Protein serine/threonine kinases

Protein serine/threonine kinases are the most frequent types of kinases that have been implicated to have a role in hearing (**Table 1**). Variants of all member genes of this group, except for *MYO3A*, cause syndromic deafness in humans (**Table 1**). In some instances, hearing loss is accompanied by ear malformations, as is the case in patients with frontometaphyseal dysplasia 2. Frontometaphyseal dysplasia 2 is caused due to variants affecting MAP3K7, and conductive or sensorineural deafness is accompanied by ear malformations [14]. For a vast majority of protein serine/threonine kinases, such as CDC42BPB, CDK8, CDK9, CDK10, CDK13, the association of hearing loss due to variants of the genes in the corresponding syndromes is based on the presence of the auditory phenotype in one or only a few individuals [15–19]. Therefore, some of these genetic variants links to human auditory malfunction may prove to be coincidental.

In a few cases, only particular types of variants of a gene may be associated with hearing loss. For example, patients with a heterozygous nonsense variant of *PRKCG* have spinocerebellar ataxia 14 with hearing loss, while patients with missense variants do not have an auditory phenotype [20]. In other instances, many individuals may be affected by hearing loss, but these only constitute up to 30% of the total patients reported to have a particular syndrome due to the corresponding gene variants. For example, Coffin-Lowry Syndrome is a disorder in which patients have mental retardation, skeletal defects, and movement disorders with or without hearing loss. It is caused as a result of *RPS6KA3* variants [21].

The variants of *MAPKAPK5* [22], *PRKCB* [23], and *BRAF* [24] have been reported to cause hearing loss in humans, but not in mice. Variants of some protein serine/threonine kinases such as *RAF1* [25] and *MAP3K20* [26] cause hearing loss in humans, and their orthologous genes have a demonstrated role in mouse audition as well [26, 27]. In other cases, importance of a gene to mammalian hearing can only be gauged due to the observed phenotype in mouse models. For example, pathogenic alleles of *Map3k1* [28, 29], *Map3k4* [30], *Pak1* [31], and *Stk11* [32] are reported to cause hearing loss in mice only. Mice with *Mapk1* deletion in the inner ear undergo noise-induced hearing loss [33]. However, deafness has not been reported as yet in humans, but patients with *MAPK1* variants have outer ear morphological defects [34].

An interesting example of a protein serine/threonine kinase is MYO3A since it has both a C-terminal motor domain and an N-terminal kinase domain. Its loss of function variants usually cause recessively inherited moderate to severe nonsyndromic hearing loss, which can be adult onset and progressive in nature [5]. One homozygous variant abolishes MYO3A kinase function, and the affected individuals have profound deafness [35]. Dominantly inherited *MYO3A* variants are very rare. Of the latter, a heterozygous missense variant affecting the kinase domain was reported to cause hearing loss in affected individuals of a German family [36]. The MYO3A kinase activity may be important for phosphorylation of its own motor domain, thus reducing motor activity and regulating protein concentration in the stereocilia [37].

Different mice models homozygous for a knock-in nonsense variant or a missense variant in the kinase domain have progressive hearing loss [38, 39], mimicking the phenotype observed in humans.

2.3 Protein tyrosine kinases, nonreceptor type

So far variants in two different genes encoding nonreceptor protein tyrosine kinases, ABL1 and BTK, have been reported to cause hearing loss in some patients with different syndromes. Variants of *ABL1* cause a syndromic disorder (**Table 1**) in which subsets of patients have outer ear abnormalities and hearing loss [40]. Recently, variants were reported in patients with a phenotype termed as *ABL1* malformation syndrome, and it was shown that hearing loss in the patients occurred due to the increased tyrosine kinase activity of the protein [41]. Variants of *BTK* have been reported to cause otitis media and hearing loss in a few patients with agammaglobulinemia, X-linked 1, a disorder of B-lymphocyte maturation [42].

3. Protein phosphatases

As compared the large number of kinases, the phosphatases comprise less than 1% of the human coding genes [43]. The phosphatase enzymes dephosphorylate target proteins at the serine or threonine residues (protein serine/threonine phosphatases), while some act on the tyrosine residues (protein tyrosine phosphatases) or both tyrosine and serine/threonine residues (dual-specificity phosphatases). The protein serine/threonine phosphatases are divided into three structurally related groups while all members of protein tyrosine phosphatases and dual-specificity phosphatases belong to one structurally related class. The, atypical protein phosphatases constitute a separate group, with structural features different from the other types [44]. In contrast to the protein kinases, research has identified far fewer protein phosphatases, which have an important role in the auditory system (**Table 1**). These enzymes are important for disparate developmental processes, and the targeted deletions of the pertinent genes in mice have revealed their contributions to the development of ear and maintenance of hearing. In some cases, although the phosphatase itself may not have been directly implicated yet in a human hearing loss disorder, variants in their substrate or docking proteins do cause deafness [45].

3.1 Atypical protein phosphatases

The atypical protein phosphatases have an N-terminal threonine phosphatase and a C-terminal tyrosine phosphatase domain [44]. EYA1 and EYA4 are two atypical protein phosphatases that are important for hearing. Variants of *EYA1* cause two allelic syndromes in humans, which include hearing loss as one of the manifestations, along with multiple outer and inner ear structural defects [46, 47]. Homozygous *Eya1* mutant mice lack ears, which suggest an essential role of the encoded protein in early development [48]. Similarly, EYA4 is essential for maintenance of hearing in humans [49, 50] and mice [51]. EYA4 is one of the very few phosphatases, variants of which cause nonsyndromic deafness in humans [49], although some of its variants also give rise to a syndromic form of deafness with dilated cardiomyopathy [50].

3.2 Dual-specificity phosphatases

Dual-specificity phosphatases can catalyze the removal of phosphates from both phosphorylated tyrosine and serine/threonine residues of the target proteins. They are structurally similar to the tyrosine phosphatase family enzymes. CDC14A is a dual-specificity phosphatase and has been shown to be absolutely necessary for hearing in both humans [52, 53] and mice [53]. Moreover, some variants cause hearing loss with immotile sperm in humans and mice [53]. Most phospho protein targets of CDC14A are unknown, though drebrin (DBE1) has been proposed to be one such protein [54]. Two other dual-specificity phosphatases, DUSP1 [55, 56] and DUSP6 [57], are important for hearing in mice. *Dusp1* knockout mouse mutants manifest a progressive hearing loss [56], perhaps due to disruption of cytokines [55]. Similarly, DUSP6 is required for ear development in mice [58]. Few patients with hypogonadotropic hypogonadism 19 with or without anosmia may have a hearing loss due to *DUSP6* variants [59].

One unusual dual-specific protein phosphatase is PTEN, which has both lipid phosphatase and dual-specific protein phosphatase activities. Although lipid dephosphorylation by PTEN is well studied, that of protein dephosphorylation is less so. However, it was shown that PTEN plays a role in ciliogenesis by phosphorylating the protein DVL2 [60]. Heterozygous knockout *Pten*$^{+/-}$ mice have inner ear abnormalities [61] while the inner ear specific homozygous knockout mice are deaf [62] and have supernumerary hair cells [63]. In humans, some patients with Cowden syndrome have a hearing loss due to *PTEN* variants [64].

3.3 Protein tyrosine phosphatases nonreceptor type

Variants of protein tyrosine phosphatase PTPN11 cause two autosomal dominant syndromes (**Table 1**) in which patients can have hearing loss with multiple other disorders including cardiovascular manifestations [65, 66]. Sometimes, hearing loss is presented as the first symptom of the syndrome [67], while other individuals exhibit only the auditory phenotype as a nonsyndromic case [68]. Studies in HEK293 cells have demonstrated that PTPN11 variants involved in human disorders affect dephosphorylation of GAB1 [69]; another protein that is important for hearing [70].

4. Conclusions and perspectives

Kinases and phosphatases serve as important regulators of cell signaling and protein function within the auditory system. Many of these enzymes are required for the maintenance of inner ear structures by regulating function of different proteins, which are known to be present in the hair cells. Not only are the malfunctions of these enzymes involved in genetic hearing loss, but many environmental factors such as exposure to loud noise and oxidative stress also activate or affect the phosphorylation pathways [71]. Due to the importance of MAPK pathway to hearing [71, 72], it is a target for design of treatment of hearing loss. Pharmacological inhibitors of phosphorylation pathways are being explored for treatment of hearing loss [2]. Inhibitors are specifically developed and administered to model organisms for stopping ototoxic effects of medicinal drugs [73]. For example, direct BRAF inhibition, by dabrafenib given orally, was demonstrated to protect mouse hearing loss induced due to cisplatin administration [74]. Intra-tympanic injections for treatment of noise-induced hearing loss in model organisms are also being explored and may open up avenues for effective localized therapies in humans as well [75]. Continued research on protein phosphorylation will yield additional information on other important kinases and phosphatases and their target proteins required for human hearing and will advance our understanding of the auditory system.

Acknowledgements

The author thanks Ayesha Imtiaz for suggesting this topic for review and her help during the initial phases of the work.

Author details

Sadaf Naz
University of the Punjab, School of Biological Sciences, Quaid-e-Azam Campus, Lahore, Pakistan

*Address all correspondence to: naz.sbs@pu.edu.pk

References

[1] Mateo Sanchez S, Freeman SD, Delacroix L, Malgrange B. The role of post-translational modifications in hearing and deafness. Cellular and Molecular Life Sciences. 2016;**73**(18):3521-3533

[2] Ardito F, Giuliani M, Perrone D, Troiano G, Lo Muzio L. The crucial role of protein phosphorylation in cell signaling and its use as targeted therapy (review). International Journal of Molecular Medicine. 2017;**40**(2):271-280

[3] Naz S, Friedman TB. Growth factor and receptor malfunctions associated with human genetic deafness. Clinical Genetics. 2020;**97**(1):138-155

[4] Kochhar A, Hildebrand MS, Smith RJ. Clinical aspects of hereditary hearing loss. Genetics in Medicine. 2007;**9**(7):393-408

[5] Walsh T, Walsh V, Vreugde S, Hertzano R, Shahin H, Haika S, et al. From flies' eyes to our ears: Mutations in a human class III myosin cause progressive nonsyndromic hearing loss DFNB30. Proceedings of the National Academy of Sciences of the United States of America. 2002;**99**(11):7518-7523

[6] Manning G, Whyte DB, Martinez R, Hunter T, Sudarsanam S. The protein kinase complement of the human genome. Science. 2002;**298**(5600):1912-1934

[7] Burglen L, Chantot-Bastaraud S, Garel C, Milh M, Touraine R, Zanni G, et al. Spectrum of pontocerebellar hypoplasia in 13 girls and boys with CASK mutations: Confirmation of a recognizable phenotype and first description of a male mosaic patient. Orphanet Journal of Rare Diseases. 2012;**7**:18

[8] Cimerman J, Waldhaus J, Harasztosi C, Duncker SV, Dettling J, Heidrych P, et al. Generation of somatic electromechanical force by outer hair cells may be influenced by prestin-CASK interaction at the basal junction with the Deiter's cell. Histochemistry and Cell Biology. 2013;**140**(2):119-135

[9] Zhu Y, Delhommel F, Cordier F, Luchow S, Mechaly A, Colcombet-Cazenave B, et al. Deciphering the unexpected binding capacity of the third PDZ domain of Whirlin to various Cochlear hair cell partners. Journal of Molecular Biology. 2020;**432**(22):5920-5937

[10] Zhai X, Liu C, Zhao B, Wang Y, Xu Z. Inactivation of cyclin-dependent kinase 5 in hair cells causes hearing loss in mice. Frontiers in Molecular Neuroscience. 2018;**11**:461

[11] Meissner LE, Macnamara EF, D'Souza P, Yang J, Vezina G, Ferreira CR, et al. DYRK1A pathogenic variants in two patients with syndromic intellectual disability and a review of the literature. Molecular Genetics & Genomic Medicine. 2020;**8**(12):e1544

[12] Nishi E, Mizuno S, Nanjo Y, Niihori T, Fukushima Y, Matsubara Y, et al. A novel heterozygous MAP2K1 mutation in a patient with Noonan syndrome with multiple lentigines. American Journal of Medical Genetics. Part A. 2015;**167A**(2):407-411

[13] Kosztyla-Hojna B, Borys J, Zdrojkowski M, Duchnowska E, Kraszewska A, Wasilewska D, et al. Phoniatric, audiological, Orodental and speech problems in a boy with cardio-Facio-cutaneous syndrome type 3 (CFC 3) due to a pathogenic variant in

MAP2K1 - case study. The Application of Clinical Genetics. 2021;**14**:389-398

[14] Le Goff C, Rogers C, Le Goff W, Pinto G, Bonnet D, Chrabieh M, et al. Heterozygous mutations in MAP3K7, encoding TGF-beta-activated kinase 1, cause Cardiospondylocarpofacial syndrome. American Journal of Human Genetics. 2016;**99**(2):407-413

[15] Chilton I, Okur V, Vitiello G, Selicorni A, Mariani M, Goldenberg A, et al. De novo heterozygous missense and loss-of-function variants in CDC42BPB are associated with a neurodevelopmental phenotype. American Journal of Medical Genetics. Part A. 2020;**182**(5):962-973

[16] Calpena E, Hervieu A, Kaserer T, Swagemakers SMA, Goos JAC, Popoola O, et al. De novo missense substitutions in the gene encoding CDK8, a regulator of the mediator complex, cause a syndromic developmental disorder. American Journal of Human Genetics. 2019;**104**(4):709-720

[17] Nishina S, Hosono K, Ishitani S, Kosaki K, Yokoi T, Yoshida T, et al. Biallelic CDK9 variants as a cause of a new multiple-malformation syndrome with retinal dystrophy mimicking the CHARGE syndrome. Journal of Human Genetics. 2021;**66**(10):1021-1027

[18] Guen VJ, Edvardson S, Fraenkel ND, Fattal-Valevski A, Jalas C, Anteby I, et al. A homozygous deleterious CDK10 mutation in a patient with agenesis of corpus callosum, retinopathy, and deafness. American Journal of Medical Genetics. Part A. 2018;**176**(1):92-98

[19] Acharya A, Raza SI, Anwar MZ, Bharadwaj T, Liaqat K, Khokhar MAS, et al. Wolfram-like syndrome with bicuspid aortic valve due to a homozygous missense variant in CDK13. Journal of Human Genetics. 2021;**66**(10):1009-1018

[20] Shirafuji T, Shimazaki H, Miyagi T, Ueyama T, Adachi N, Tanaka S, et al. Spinocerebellar ataxia type 14 caused by a nonsense mutation in the PRKCG gene. Molecular and Cellular Neurosciences. 2019;**98**:46-53

[21] Pereira PM, Schneider A, Pannetier S, Heron D, Hanauer A. Coffin-Lowry syndrome. European Journal of Human Genetics. 2010;**18**(6):627-633

[22] Horn D, Fernandez-Nunez E, Gomez-Carmona R, Rivera-Barahona A, Nevado J, Schwartzmann S, et al. Biallelic truncating variants in MAPKAPK5 cause a new developmental disorder involving neurological, cardiac, and facial anomalies combined with synpolydactyly. Genetics in Medicine. 2021;**23**(4):679-688

[23] Martin-Sierra C, Requena T, Frejo L, Price SD, Gallego-Martinez A, Batuecas-Caletrio A, et al. A novel missense variant in PRKCB segregates low-frequency hearing loss in an autosomal dominant family with Meniere's disease. Human Molecular Genetics. 2016;**25**(16):3407-3415

[24] Schulz AL, Albrecht B, Arici C, van der Burgt I, Buske A, Gillessen-Kaesbach G, et al. Mutation and phenotypic spectrum in patients with cardio-facio-cutaneous and Costello syndrome. Clinical Genetics. 2008;**73**(1):62-70

[25] Pandit B, Sarkozy A, Pennacchio LA, Carta C, Oishi K, Martinelli S, et al. Gain-of-function RAF1 mutations cause Noonan and LEOPARD syndromes with hypertrophic cardiomyopathy. Nature Genetics. 2007;**39**(8):1007-1012

[26] Spielmann M, Kakar N, Tayebi N, Leettola C, Nurnberg G, Sowada N,

et al. Exome sequencing and CRISPR/Cas genome editing identify mutations of ZAK as a cause of limb defects in humans and mice. Genome Research. 2016;**26**(2):183-191

[27] de Iriarte RR, Magarinos M, Pfeiffer V, Rapp UR, Varela-Nieto I. C-Raf deficiency leads to hearing loss and increased noise susceptibility. Cellular and Molecular Life Sciences. 2015;**72**(20):3983-3998

[28] Parker A, Cross SH, Jackson IJ, Hardisty-Hughes R, Morse S, Nicholson G, et al. The goya mouse mutant reveals distinct newly identified roles for MAP3K1 in the development and survival of cochlear sensory hair cells. Disease Models & Mechanisms. 2015;**8**(12):1555-1568

[29] Yousaf R, Meng Q, Hufnagel RB, Xia Y, Puligilla C, Ahmed ZM, et al. MAP3K1 function is essential for cytoarchitecture of the mouse organ of Corti and survival of auditory hair cells. Disease Models & Mechanisms. 2015;**8**(12):1543-1553

[30] Haque K, Pandey AK, Zheng HW, Riazuddin S, Sha SH, Puligilla C. MEKK4 signaling regulates sensory cell development and function in the mouse inner ear. The Journal of Neuroscience. 2016;**36**(4):1347-1361

[31] Cheng C, Hou Y, Zhang Z, Wang Y, Lu L, Zhang L, et al. Disruption of the autism-related gene Pak1 causes stereocilia disorganization, hair cell loss, and deafness in mice. Journal of Genetics and Genomics. 2021;**48**(4):324-332

[32] Men Y, Zhang A, Li H, Zhang T, Jin Y, Zhang J, et al. LKB1 is required for the development and maintenance of Stereocilia in inner ear hair cells in mice. PLoS One. 2015;**10**(8):e0135841

[33] Kurioka T, Matsunobu T, Satoh Y, Niwa K, Endo S, Fujioka M, et al. ERK2 mediates inner hair cell survival and decreases susceptibility to noise-induced hearing loss. Scientific Reports. 2015;**5**:16839

[34] Motta M, Pannone L, Pantaleoni F, Bocchinfuso G, Radio FC, Cecchetti S, et al. Enhanced MAPK1 function causes a neurodevelopmental disorder within the RASopathy clinical Spectrum. American Journal of Human Genetics. 2020;**107**(3):499-513

[35] Souissi A, Abdelmalek Driss D, Chakchouk I, Ben Said M, Ben Ayed I, Mosrati MA, et al. Molecular insights into MYO3A kinase domain variants explain variability in both severity and progression of DFNB30 hearing impairment. Journal of Biomolecular Structure & Dynamics. 2021;**20**(1):1-12

[36] Doll J, Hofrichter MAH, Bahena P, Heihoff A, Segebarth D, Muller T, et al. A novel missense variant in MYO3A is associated with autosomal dominant high-frequency hearing loss in a German family. Molecular Genetics & Genomic Medicine. 2020;**8**(8):e1343

[37] Quintero OA, Unrath WC, Stevens SM Jr, Manor U, Kachar B, Yengo CM. Myosin 3A kinase activity is regulated by phosphorylation of the kinase domain activation loop. The Journal of Biological Chemistry. 2013;**288**(52):37126-37137

[38] Li P, Wen Z, Zhang G, Zhang A, Fu X, Gao J. Knock-In mice with Myo3a Y137C mutation displayed progressive hearing loss and hair cell degeneration in the inner ear. Neural Plasticity. 2018;**2018**:4372913

[39] Walsh VL, Raviv D, Dror AA, Shahin H, Walsh T, Kanaan MN, et al. A mouse model for human hearing loss DFNB30 due to loss of function of myosin IIIA. Mammalian Genome. 2011;**22**(3-4):170-177

[40] Chen CA, Crutcher E, Gill H, Nelson TN, Robak LA, Jongmans MCJ, et al. The expanding clinical phenotype of germline ABL1-associated congenital heart defects and skeletal malformations syndrome. Human Mutation. 2020;**41**(10):1738-1744

[41] Blakes AJM, Gaul E, Lam W, Shannon N, Knapp KM, Bicknell LS, et al. Pathogenic variants causing ABL1 malformation syndrome cluster in a myristoyl-binding pocket and increase tyrosine kinase activity. European Journal of Human Genetics. 2021;**29**(4):593-603

[42] Berlucchi M, Soresina A, Redaelli De Zinis LO, Valetti L, Valotti R, Lougaris V, et al. Sensorineural hearing loss in primary antibody deficiency disorders. The Journal of Pediatrics. 2008;**153**(2):293-296

[43] Chen MJ, Dixon JE, Manning G. Genomics and evolution of protein phosphatases. Science Signaling. 2017;**10**(474):eaag1796

[44] Sadatomi D, Tanimura S, Ozaki K, Takeda K. Atypical protein phosphatases: Emerging players in cellular signaling. International Journal of Molecular Sciences. 2013;**14**(3):4596-4612

[45] Ferrar T, Chamousset D, De Wever V, Nimick M, Andersen J, Trinkle-Mulcahy L, et al. Taperin (c9orf75), a mutated gene in nonsyndromic deafness, encodes a vertebrate specific, nuclear localized protein phosphatase one alpha (PP1alpha) docking protein. Biology Open. 2012;**1**(2):128-139

[46] Abdelhak S, Kalatzis V, Heilig R, Compain S, Samson D, Vincent C, et al. A human homologue of the drosophila eyes absent gene underlies branchio-Oto-renal (BOR) syndrome and identifies a novel gene family. Nature Genetics. 1997;**15**(2):157-164

[47] Vincent C, Kalatzis V, Abdelhak S, Chaib H, Compain S, Helias J, et al. BOR and BO syndromes are allelic defects of EYA1. European Journal of Human Genetics. 1997;**5**(4):242-246

[48] Xu PX, Adams J, Peters H, Brown MC, Heaney S, Maas R. Eya1-deficient mice lack ears and kidneys and show abnormal apoptosis of organ primordia. Nature Genetics. 1999;**23**(1):113-117

[49] Wayne S, Robertson NG, DeClau F, Chen N, Verhoeven K, Prasad S, et al. Mutations in the transcriptional activator EYA4 cause late-onset deafness at the DFNA10 locus. Human Molecular Genetics. 2001;**10**(3):195-200

[50] Schonberger J, Wang L, Shin JT, Kim SD, Depreux FF, Zhu H, et al. Mutation in the transcriptional coactivator EYA4 causes dilated cardiomyopathy and sensorineural hearing loss. Nature Genetics. 2005;**37**(4):418-422

[51] Depreux FF, Darrow K, Conner DA, Eavey RD, Liberman MC, Seidman CE, et al. Eya4-deficient mice are a model for heritable otitis media. The Journal of Clinical Investigation. 2008;**118**(2):651-658

[52] Delmaghani S, Aghaie A, Bouyacoub Y, El Hachmi H, Bonnet C, Riahi Z, et al. Mutations in CDC14A, encoding a protein phosphatase involved in hair cell Ciliogenesis, cause autosomal-recessive severe to profound deafness. American Journal of Human Genetics. 2016;**98**(6):1266-1270

[53] Imtiaz A, Belyantseva IA, Beirl AJ, Fenollar-Ferrer C, Bashir R, Bukhari I, et al. CDC14A phosphatase is essential for hearing and male fertility in mouse and human. Human Molecular Genetics. 2018;**27**(5):780-798

[54] Uddin B, Partscht P, Chen NP, Neuner A, Weiss M, Hardt R, et al. The human phosphatase CDC14A modulates primary cilium length by regulating centrosomal actin nucleation. EMBO Reports. 2019;**20**(1):e46544

[55] Bermudez-Munoz JM, Celaya AM, Garcia-Mato A, Munoz-Espin D, Rodriguez-de la Rosa L, Serrano M, et al. Dual-specificity phosphatase 1 (DUSP1) has a central role in redox homeostasis and inflammation in the mouse cochlea. Antioxidants (Basel). 2021;**10**(9):1351

[56] Celaya AM, Sanchez-Perez I, Bermudez-Munoz JM, Rodriguez-de la Rosa L, Pintado-Berninches L, Perona R, et al. Deficit of mitogen-activated protein kinase phosphatase 1 (DUSP1) accelerates progressive hearing loss. eLife. 2019;**8**:e39159

[57] Li C, Scott DA, Hatch E, Tian X, Mansour SL. Dusp6 (Mkp3) is a negative feedback regulator of FGF-stimulated ERK signaling during mouse development. Development. 2007;**134**(1):167-176

[58] Urness LD, Li C, Wang X, Mansour SL. Expression of ERK signaling inhibitors Dusp6, Dusp7, and Dusp9 during mouse ear development. Developmental Dynamics. 2008;**237**(1):163-169

[59] Miraoui H, Dwyer AA, Sykiotis GP, Plummer L, Chung W, Feng B, et al. Mutations in FGF17, IL17RD, DUSP6, SPRY4, and FLRT3 are identified in individuals with congenital hypogonadotropic hypogonadism. American Journal of Human Genetics. 2013;**92**(5):725-743

[60] Shnitsar I, Bashkurov M, Masson GR, Ogunjimi AA, Mosessian S, Cabeza EA, et al. PTEN regulates cilia through Dishevelled. Nature Communications. 2015;**6**:8388

[61] Dong Y, Sui L, Yamaguchi F, Kamitori K, Hirata Y, Hossain MA, et al. Phosphatase and tensin homolog deleted on chromosome 10 regulates sensory cell proliferation and differentiation of hair bundles in the mammalian cochlea. Neuroscience. 2010;**170**(4):1304-1313

[62] Kim HJ, Woo HM, Ryu J, Bok J, Kim JW, Choi SB, et al. Conditional deletion of pten leads to defects in nerve innervation and neuronal survival in inner ear development. PLoS One. 2013;**8**(2):e55609

[63] Sun C, Zhao J, Jin Y, Hou C, Zong W, Lu T, et al. PTEN regulation of the proliferation and differentiation of auditory progenitors through the PTEN/PI3K/Akt-signaling pathway in mice. Neuroreport. 2014;**25**(3):177-183

[64] Taylor A, Delon I, Allinson K, Trotman J, Liu H, Abbs S, et al. Malignant peripheral nerve sheath tumor in cowden syndrome: A first report. Journal of Neuropathology and Experimental Neurology. 2015;**74**(4):288-292

[65] Yoshida R, Nagai T, Hasegawa T, Kinoshita E, Tanaka T, Ogata T. Two novel and one recurrent PTPN11 mutations in LEOPARD syndrome. American Journal of Medical Genetics. Part A. 2004;**130A**(4):432-434

[66] Tartaglia M, Mehler EL, Goldberg R, Zampino G, Brunner HG, Kremer H, et al. Mutations in PTPN11, encoding the protein tyrosine phosphatase SHP-2, cause Noonan syndrome. Nature Genetics. 2001;**29**(4):465-468

[67] Gao X, Huang SS, Qiu SW, Su Y, Wang WQ, Xu HY, et al. Congenital sensorineural hearing loss as the initial presentation of PTPN11-associated

Noonan syndrome with multiple lentigines or Noonan syndrome: Clinical features and underlying mechanisms. Journal of Medical Genetics. 2021;**58**(7):465-474

[68] Bademci G, Cengiz FB, Foster Ii J, Duman D, Sennaroglu L, Diaz-Horta O, et al. Variations in multiple syndromic deafness genes mimic non-syndromic hearing loss. Scientific Reports. 2016;**6**:31622

[69] Edouard T, Combier JP, Nedelec A, Bel-Vialar S, Metrich M, Conte-Auriol F, et al. Functional effects of PTPN11 (SHP2) mutations causing LEOPARD syndrome on epidermal growth factor-induced phosphoinositide 3-kinase/AKT/glycogen synthase kinase 3beta signaling. Molecular and Cellular Biology. 2010;**30**(10):2498-2507

[70] Yousaf R, Ahmed ZM, Giese AP, Morell RJ, Lagziel A, Dabdoub A, et al. Modifier variant of METTL13 suppresses human GAB1-associated profound deafness. The Journal of Clinical Investigation. 2018;**128**(4):1509-1522

[71] Liu Y, Wei M, Mao X, Chen T, Lin P, Wang W. Key signaling pathways regulate the development and survival of auditory hair cells. Neural Plasticity. 2021;**2021**:5522717

[72] Alagramam KN, Stepanyan R, Jamesdaniel S, Chen DH, Davis RR. Noise exposure immediately activates cochlear mitogen-activated protein kinase signaling. Noise & Health. 2014;**16**(73):400-409

[73] Hazlitt RA, Teitz T, Bonga JD, Fang J, Diao S, Iconaru L, et al. Development of second-generation CDK2 inhibitors for the prevention of cisplatin-induced hearing loss. Journal of Medicinal Chemistry. 2018;**61**(17):7700-7709

[74] Ingersoll MA, Malloy EA, Caster LE, Holland EM, Xu Z, Zallocchi M, et al. BRAF inhibition protects against hearing loss in mice. Science Advances. 2020;**6**(49):eabd0561

[75] Rybak LP, Dhukhwa A, Mukherjea D, Ramkumar V. Local drug delivery for prevention of hearing loss. Frontiers in Cellular Neuroscience. 2019;**13**:300

Section 4

Improved Treatments for Hearing Loss

Chapter 8

Issues in Creation of Bio-Compatible Cochlear Signal: Towards a New Generation of Cochlear Prosthetic Devices

Wlodzimierz ("Vlad") Wojcik

Abstract

A model of a fully functional cochlear prosthesis is presented here, simplified by taking into account only those evolutionary features of natural cochleae that contribute to their functionality. The proposed prosthetic device generates a bio-compatible digital signal which can be fed to the cochlear nerve. Subsequently, analysis of cochlear nerve signals is offered, both natural and artificial. To that end a number of mathematical theorems are formulated, proven, and then used to demonstrate that signals obtained from our prosthetic device are useful towards auditory pattern recognition, audio location, and even speech comprehension, as well as understanding and enjoyment of music.

Keywords: audio pattern recognition, auditory pathway, auditory cilia, cochlea, cochlear model, cochlear nerve signal, cochlear prostheses, mechanoreceptors

1. Introduction

Imagine a deaf patient who lost her outer, middle, and inner ears through disease or injury. The remaining parts of her auditory pathway (cochlear nerve, cochlear nucleus, superior olive, lateral lemniscus, inferior colliculus, medial geniculate body, and auditory cortex) are intact. Although profoundly deaf, the patient is not hopeless. She expects us to fit her with two electronic devices that would feed suitable signals to her cochlear nerves, thus allowing her to hear again.

The current cochlear implant devices are exceedingly basic: they normally assist or compensate for certain malfunctions of damaged parts of middle or inner ear (auditory cells, tectorial membrane, etc.) but offer only crude restorative signals spanning approx. 10 channels. To appreciate the inadequacy of the current state-of-the-art, the reader might want to peruse simulations at [1].

In contrast, healthy human cochlear nerve consists of approx. 30,000 neural axons, with almost every axon conveying one channel of a signal. Humans do not hold any records in this regard: feline cochlear nerves contain approx. 50,000 axon fibers. The information traveling through neural axons is digital in nature, due to all-or-nothing neural axon hillock operation when generating signal. No wonder then that the problem of refining cochlear implants catches interest of some computer scientists.

Formation of the complete multi-channel, representative signal adhering to the biological cochlear nerve signal protocol is a daunting task, requiring deep understanding of the workings of outer, middle, and inner ears, which participate in the signal generation process, as well as the workings of organs in the auditory pathway, which receive and interpret these signals. While the functionality of ear organs is relatively well understood, the same cannot be said about the organs higher up the auditory pathway. We shed some light here on their functionality.

The biologists and physicians instill in us the awe for the complexity of biological organs. Ears are such organs. Outer ears are sound channeling and amplification devices, processing sound waves traveling through air. Middle ears are mechanical in nature: their tiny ossicles (malleus, incus, and stapes) controlled by equally tiny muscles amplify weak signals or dampen strong signals before conveying them to inner ear. In this way the inner ear is protected. Finally, inner ears are wonders of electromechanical and electrochemical precision, governed by the laws of fluid dynamics, etc.

Our goal is to build an electronic device creating a fully restorative cochlear signal without entering too deep into details of functionality of biological ears. We argue that our ears are unnecessarily complex for their function. They emerged through the process of evolution, not intelligent design. That evolutionary process consists of introducing random changes into the genotype (via crossover and mutation) and then ensuring of survival of the fittest individuals via natural selection. In this way only deleterious genetic changes are eliminated. Neutral changes are allowed to remain, thus unnecessarily increasing the complexity of emerging systems.

Biological textbooks offer many examples of such unnecessary complications introduced by the evolutionary process: consider the path of laryngeal nerve, allowing the brain to control the larynx. The nerve's inferior (recurrent) branch, innervating larynx muscles, is unnecessarily long: it descends from the brain into the thorax only then to return to the larynx. In medical textbooks it is frequently cited as an evidence of evolution: in giraffes this extra length can be measured in meters! This feature is a vestige of an evolutionary process—in fish throats and gills are in immediate vicinity so this detour did not exist when fish were the most complex animals.

Another example could be the structure of an eye. Human retina has a blind spot; also, tiny blood vessels supplying blood to the retina are positioned in front of it, rather than behind it, thus occluding some sensory cells (rods and cones). Such clumsy "design blunder" can only evolve through a process of mutations and natural selection. To compensate for that "blunder" the brain's visual cortex had to evolve unnecessary complexity. We have already decoded the fundamental workings of the visual cortex [2, 3]; here the same methodology is used to attack the problem of signal processing for auditory perception.

The complexity of the central nervous system (CNS) to a large degree is due to existence of structures compensating for its earlier structural inefficiencies. The difficulty in figuring out the inner workings of CNS stems from the fact that the biologists must study with equal diligence all parts of the CNS: those essential and those secondary to its functionality. They have no choice there: to distinguish between the roles of these parts is to understand the CNS functionality.

This multi-disciplinary chapter consists of two parts:

We start by presenting a simplified but functionally complete model of our auditory perception, together with an electronic model of a device capable of providing restorative signal to the cochlear nerve, thus suggesting a new generation of cochlear prostheses. This functional description is targeted at electronic engineers who may have little biological background but will be tasked with creation of electronic circuits producing suitable e-cochlear signals.

Following that we demonstrate mathematically that signals so obtained carry information useful to the healthy part of the auditory pathway to perform the well-understood functions of audio location, as well as the more complex functions of audio pattern recognition and may even give rise to the subjective pleasure of music, so enjoyed by healthy humans. This section is written with some mathematical rigor.

2. The nature of auditory perception

Departing from the traditional phase-based or frequency-based models of cochlear and vestibular signals we offer simpler, unified, and biologically inspired insights that rely on massive parallelism, needed for real time auditory pattern recognition. Our signal analysis is also applicable to vestibular signals, used to balance body equilibrium and posture, as well as to stabilize retinal image.

To justify our approach to auditory perception modeling consider a hare hearing a noise: it uses its audio signal to detect a possible predator approaching, in order to take a prompt evasive action. Our hare uses its auditory pattern recognition skills live, as soon as it starts hearing the noise; this is necessary for hare's survival.

Luckily for all of us (hares included) the signals we perceive are causal. A signal $f(t)$ is causal, iff

$$f(t) = 0 \text{ for all } t < 0 \tag{1}$$

This work deals with causal signals, in the above sense.

To cope with causal signals, we build causal systems. An output $y(t_0)$ of a causal system at a given time t_0 depends only on its causal input $x(t)$, for all $t \le t_0$. We create causal systems by building their causal models first.

The simplest (trivial!) causal system can be modeled as follows:

Given an input signal $x(t)$ for $0 \le t \le t_0$, we may create a causal model that copies the input signal to its output, that is, produces $y(t) = x(t)$. A memory-less causal system using such a trivial model is pretty much useless: it cannot understand the signal it processes.

We strive to create systems that use causal models in anticipatory fashion, that is, intending to forecast (within desired accuracy and meeting specific time deadlines) the input signal $x(t_1)$ at some future time $t_1 > t_0$ on the basis of a known input $x(t)$ for $0 \le t \le t_0$. For that we need an intelligent system.

Indeed, this is the essence of *intelligence* demanded of a system meeting challenges of its environment. A system is intelligent if it is capable of forecasting reliably enough its future causal input signals, while meeting forecasting deadlines. The longer forecast horizon and the better accuracy of prediction, the higher is the intelligence of such a system.

Example: Our hare hearing a noise may estimate the proximity, the direction, and speed of an approaching predator, and then timely identify and execute suitable evasive action. A hare capable of routinely saving its skin in this way is considered intelligent, that is, well adapted to its environment. To be so adapted the hare need not only to be versed in auditory perception, but also capable of real-time execution of its algorithms.

Example: Humans understand and like music. What is it exactly that we like?

When we say that we understand a causal signal we mean that we perceive patterns in it, and, using them, we are capable of building a predictive model of the signal. In this chapter we preoccupy ourselves with audio signals. Some of them we perceive as noise, some of them as music. How can we tell the difference? Or, is there a difference?

Following the logic just presented we say that we understand a particular audio signal, if we can forecast future signal values with satisfactory accuracy within some time horizon. To understand an audio signal means to have a useful model of it. We feel pleasure when we can accomplish this, and term such signal music (or speech, etc.) Other signals are termed noise. Additional pleasure is instinctively drawn from the realization that we are coping successfully with the challenges of our environment, and in particular, when listening to music that we are not in any danger regardless of the success or failure of our predictions; and so, we can hone our predictive skills in complete safety by listening to music, perhaps repeatedly.

Observe further that a previously taped "musical" signal can still be perceived as "noise" if reproduced at modified speed, or perhaps played backwards, thus making real-time forecasting impossible. This reinforces our view that the signal counts only as "music" if we can understand it, that is, identify patterns within it, use these patterns for forecasting its future passages while executing in real time the entire computation of forecasts, before the actual signals arrive. That successful verification of hearing our forecasts coinciding with reality as time advances (within "reasonable" tolerances) we call enjoyment of music or understanding of speech – at least in terms of adherence to relevant grammatical rules.

The larger goals of our research are twofold: (1) to further the understanding of the working of the CNS including human brain and (2) to learn how to build smarter devices, capable of interfacing with our CNS. Here we pursue both goals, using the methodology previously successful in decoding fundamentals of visual signal processing [2, 3]. Drawing on biological inspirations we limit our use of math tools to set theory and theory of metric spaces. After all, even simple animals seem to execute in timely fashion the forecasting models appropriate to their environmental niches. We doubt that simple animals have sufficient computing skills to execute complex math in real-time. In the spirit of Occam's razor, we value simplicity. Simple models can be executed fast. When it comes to survival, speed counts!

Although the focus of this chapter is on cochlear signal processing, it is worth noting that all nerve signals are similar in structure and this similarity is of immediate practical interest in vestibular nerve signal processing. The vestibular system is responsible for sensing body equilibrium and posture, as well as for stabilizing eyeballs when we move our heads (a *Steadicam* function) [4–7].

3. Basic model of auditory perception

For the purposes of this chapter, we would like to offer a simplified engineering model of human auditory perception. At the outset we beg for indulgence of our biologically trained readers: detailed descriptions of this system are available elsewhere [8], including other chapters of this book.

Our description focuses on features of the system in need of further explanation, namely those of interpretation of signals by the auditory cortex. We limit our description of anatomy to essential features only.

The brain's auditory pathway consists of *cochlear nucleus*, *superior olive*, *lateral lemniscus*, *inferior colliculus*, *medial geniculate body*, *thalamus*, and terminating at *auditory cortex*.

Vigorous research activity is aimed at understanding the functionality of these brain nuclei by studying their neural structure. We propose a different approach, which we tested successfully when studying the functionality of human vision system [2, 3]. As pointed out already, we are convinced that these brain nuclei are exceedingly complex, as they contain structures essential to their function as well as those merely vestigial to the evolutionary process. To discern between those two kinds is not possible without understanding the functionality of the auditory pathway, which is the very goal of this research effort.

Facing this circular conundrum, we prefer another investigative approach: given the information traveling via cochlear nerve we attempt to deduce the structure and functionality of an abstract computer needed to account for auditory perception we (humans) experience. We depart from the assumption that intelligence must be wet or carbon-based; for us these are just details of a particular implementation. We prefer silicon.

Figure 1 depicts the schematic anatomy of the human ear. We mention in passing the well-known facts: the acoustic signal, that is, the air-pressure wave, traveling through the external auditory canal impedes on tympanic membrane, a.k.a. eardrum, causing it to vibrate.

The tiny bones of the middle ear (malleus, incus, and stapes) convey the mechanical vibrations of the eardrum to the cochlea where the sound perception begins.

The cochlea is a chamber filled with fluids (called perilymph and endolymph), which are in turn induced to vibrate. In engineering terms, the cochlea acts as an attenuating waveguide. It is most permeable to low frequencies, while strongly attenuating high frequencies.

Human ear can at best discern frequencies within the 20 Hz–20 kHz range. Other animals can hear within different frequency ranges, but the principle of operation of their cochleae remains the same: high frequencies are perceived only in the cochlear region close to the stapes, middle frequencies penetrate deeper, but only low

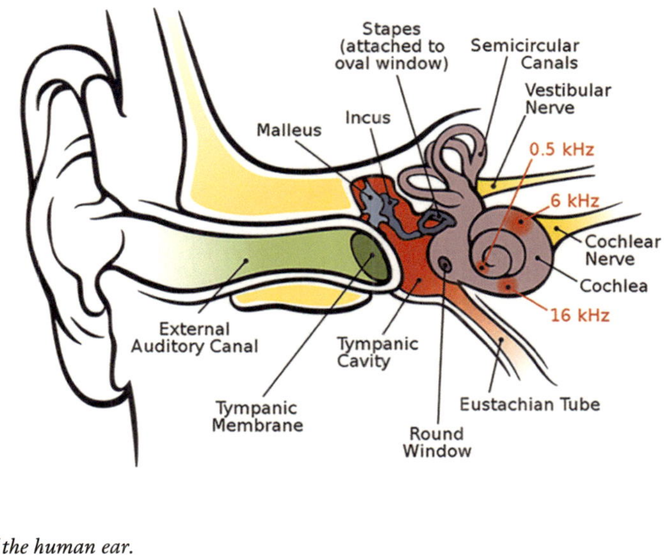

Figure 1.
Basic anatomy of the human ear.

frequencies can travel though entire cochlea. This distribution of frequency sensitivity along the length of the cochlea is referred to as *tonotopy*.

As the cochlear perilymph vibrates, it actuates the *auditory cilia*, that is, "hairs" of the "hair cells," which convert these vibrations into electrical signals. These signals are then communicated (via *neurotransmitters*) to the nerve cells of the cochlear nerve, which passes the signals to the brain.

The hair cells are organized into the *organ of Corti*, shown in the cochlear cross-section of **Figure 2**.

We omit here again many details of primary interest to anatomists, while focusing mainly on the cochlear duct called *scala media* (shown in green in **Figure 2**). It is filled with *endolymph* and contains the organ of Corti, attached to the *basilar membrane*, being one of the walls of scala media.

Organ of Corti contains large number of mechanoreceptors, called *auditory cells*. Each auditory cell is equipped with 100–150 whiskers, called *auditory cilia*, all bathed by vibrating endolymph. Some of the longer cilia are attached to the *tectorial membrane*. Both basilar and tectorial membranes also vibrate with the endolymph.

Figure 3 shows the rudimentary schematics of an auditory cell.

At resting state (no sound wave) the auditory cell body maintains certain equilibrium, measured in terms of an electrochemical potential of cell body interior. It sends then no signal to its cochlear neuron.

The sound vibrations of the endolymph in scala media impact on the single cilium shown causing it to bend sideways.

Deflection of the cilium in one direction causes excitatory increase of potential inside cell body. When that potential reaches a certain threshold level, called *action potential*, the cell issues into its synapse a certain amount of a specific neurotransmitter, which in turn causes electric signal to travel through the cochlear neuron.

Deflection of the cilium in opposite direction has inhibitory effect on cell body potential, thus silencing the cell.

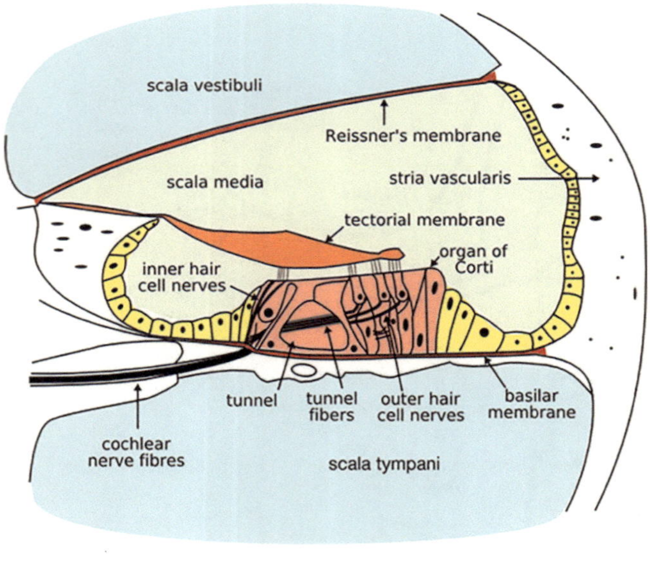

Figure 2.
Cochlear cross-section showing the organ of Corti.

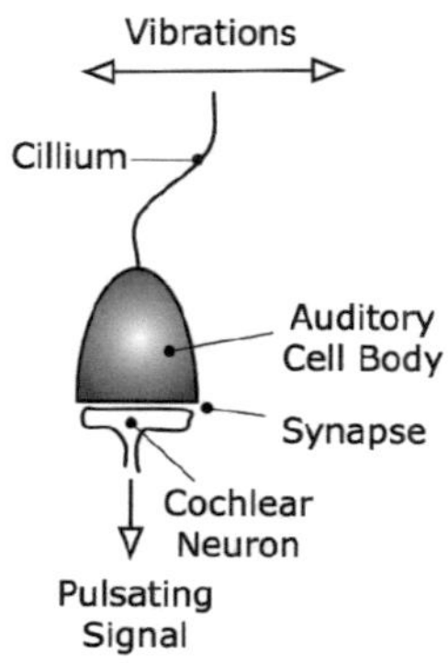

Figure 3.
Rudimentary schematics of an auditory cell.

In short, responses to vibration of the endolymph in scala media of the organ of Corti cause periodic changes in the potential of the auditory cell, thus causing a series of pulses travel through the *axon* of a cochlear neuron (i.e., *cochlear nerve fiber*) associated with that auditory cell.

The cochlear nerve is a bundle of axons of cochlear neurons. Consequently, signals traveling through cochlear nerve constitute simultaneous groups of series of pulses, each series being transmitted sequentially by a particular fiber of the nerve.

Given that the cochlea acts as non-linear waveguide, attenuating various frequencies differently, every place along its length experiences different sound pattern. For the purpose of pattern recognition, it would then be best if a number of mechanoreceptors (hair cells) were placed in exactly the same cochlear location.

However, every hair cell has finite dimensions, so it is impossible to place a number of them in the same location. Nature had no choice but to distribute them along the organ of Corti. No wonder then that different hair cells respond differently to various frequencies. All these cells are anatomically identical; their varying responses result from being exposed to different vibrations of the endolymph in their particular locations. This is the essence of tonotopy.

Nature has done everything possible to reduce the consequences of building the organ of Corti, populated by hair cells, as having non-zero dimensions, by filling the inner ear with liquid. The speed of sound waves in liquids is an order of magnitude higher that in gases. The relationship between the wavelength λ and the sound frequency f is $\lambda = v/f$, where v is the speed of sound in each of these media. From this it follows that for a given frequency f the sound wavelength in liquid is much longer than in gas, thus reducing the relative consequence of distribution of hair cells along the organ of Corti. The auditory cilia of these cells vibrate much more in sync when bathed by a liquid than they would if they were in gas. Furthermore, the inner ear is encased in the hardest bone found in a human body. This arrangement maximizes the agitation of cilia, by forcing the liquid to vibrate along the cochlea, and so perpendicularly to the cilia.

High audio acuity requires large numbers of auditory cilia, and so a larger organ of Corti in a longer cochlea. No wonder then that in simpler animals the cochleae are straight, while more complex animals have their cochleae coiled. It all has to do with the problem of packing of an elongated cochlea into a small cranial cavity within an exceptionally hard bone.

Loudness is a subjective quality of sound that is an attribute of auditory perception. We all classify sounds on some scale ranging from "quiet" to "loud." However, sound experience is a creation of our brain, a correlate with a physical phenomenon (a sound wave) impacting on our ears. Sound waves can be measured in terms of physical values like power, amplitude, frequency, sound pressure, etc.

Given that our eardrums react to sound pressure, it seems logical to correlate loudness with sound pressure. This relationship, depicted in **Figure 4**, is particularly dependent on frequency. We can easily perceive relatively weak sound waves, as long as their frequencies lie within an interval of 1–4 kHz, this being the predominant frequency range of human speech. Sound waves outside of that interval (both of higher and lower frequencies) must be substantially stronger to be perceived as equally loud. This non-linearity arises due to the inertia of the mechanical parts of our ears (eardrums, malleus, incus, and stapes) as well as the inertia and drag of the auditory cilia against the surrounding liquid. Our novel cochlear prostheses need to account for all these nonlinearities.

To outline our modeling methodology, consider an arbitrary signal (shown in blue), traveling through endolymph and impacting on an auditory cilium of a hair cell, depicted in **Figure 5**.

That cell has an action potential $a_p = 0.25$ units and generates a packet of rectangular pulses (shown in red) inscribed within the endolymph pressure wave as observed at the cell location. Its neighboring cells may have action potentials set at different values, and together they describe the pressure wave with some accuracy. Note that this description is not exact, as one would need (mathematically speaking) an infinite number of cells at the very same location in scala media, all with different action potentials (forming a continuum) to describe the signal exactly. In that sense the pressure wave could be seen as curve enveloping all possible inscribed square pulse signals.

The illustration in **Figure 5** depicts a wave of sufficiently low frequency, so that the relevant auditory cell is able to inscribe a square pulse into each peak of the audio

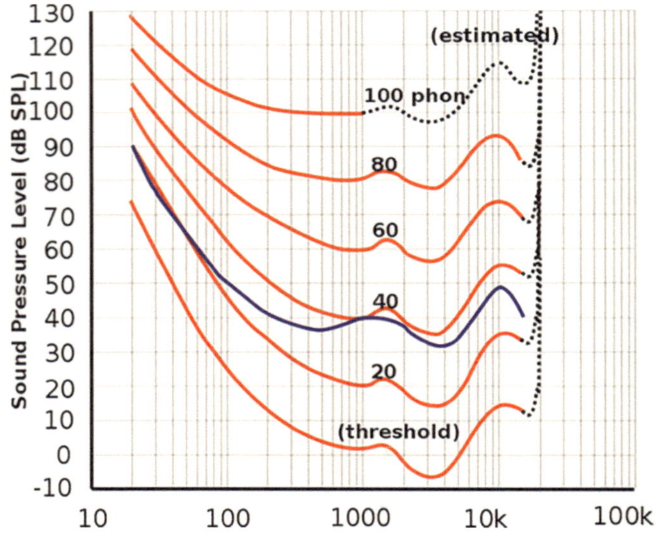

Figure 4.
Contours of equal loudness (red) as functions of frequency (Hz), ISO 226:2003 revision. Older ISO standard for 40-phon shown in blue.

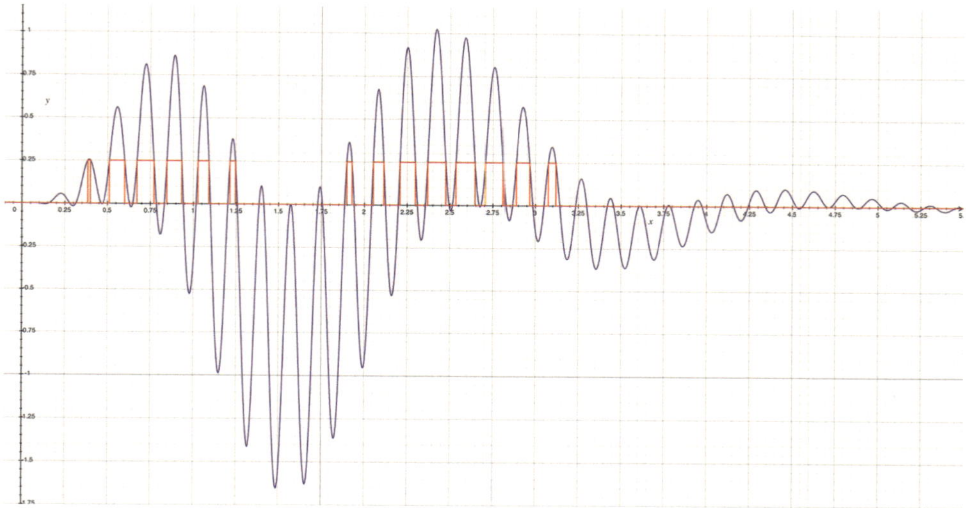

Figure 5.
Hair cell with action potential $a_p = 0.25$ inscribes a square-wave signal (red) within a sample pressure wave (blue) of an endolymph.

wave. Not all audio cells are capable of such behavior. Due to their inertia, they need time to adjust their electrochemical potential levels. An inhibited call will need more time to bring its potential to the action level than a cell that was in a neutral state. After firing a pulse each cell requires certain amount of time to bring itself into the state of readiness to fire again.

The net result of this is that the cells do not always faithfully inscribe their pulses into the acoustic wave, although the firing of their pulses is stimulated by that wave. The inertia of all cells is similar and so they generate pulses of similar frequency characteristics. It is their location in the cochlea and their connections to relevant axons of the cochlear nerve that causes us to perceive varying pitch.

The emerging bundle of signals formed in this way, traveling along the cochlear nerve, carries to the auditory cortex the information about the ambient sound wave.

Specifically, there is only a finite number of cells with different action potentials in a particular region. That region being small, we can assume that all of them respond in sync to the same pressure wave. Our model deals therefore with bundles of square pulse approximations of the sound wave. According to the Shannon-Hartley theorem [9, 10] these approximations can be still exact even for a finite number of hair cells used, provided that their stimulating signal lies within certain harmonic limitations.

The frequency region of 20 Hz–20 kHz is not such limitation, as it only describes limits of the audible frequency response curve for human hair cells. Acoustic signals outside this range are merely inaudible but they do exist. Certainly, some harmonic limitations of an acoustic signal exist. Given that wave energy is proportional to the wave frequency, there must be some limit to the number of frequency components of a given audio signal for the signal to carry finite energy. We inhabit a universe filled with signals of finite energies—because of that we can exist.

Let us take a closer look at square pulse signals of finite length. There is a number of possible descriptions of a signal s(t) consisting of n pulses:

$$s(t) = \langle t_0, t_1, t_2, t_3, \dots t_{2n-1} \rangle \tag{2}$$

where < •, •, ... • > is a tuple of 2n values listed in strictly ascending order, that is, for every pair of values t_i, t_k such that $i < k$ we have $t_i < t_k$. The time values with an even index define the beginning of a pulse, the times with odd index represent the end of a pulse.

Alternatively, we can represent signal s(t) as a set of mutually exclusive time-line intervals:

$$s(t) = \{[t_0, t_1), [t_2, t_3), \ldots, [t_{n-2}, t_{n-1})\} \tag{3}$$

Using this description signal values for arbitrary t can be calculated as follows:

$$s(t) = \begin{cases} a_p \text{ for } t_i \leq t < t_{i+1} \text{ where i is even;} \\ 0 \text{ for } t_i < t \leq t_{i+1} \text{ where i is odd.} \end{cases} \tag{4}$$

In fact, we will deal mostly with normalized signals, that is, assuming values 0 and 1. Such signals can be obtained by dividing the above pulse signal by its action potential, viz. $s(t)/a_p$ yielding:

$$s(t) = \begin{cases} 1 \text{ for } t_i \leq t < t_{i+1} \text{ where i is even;} \\ 0 \text{ for } t_i < t \leq t_{i+1} \text{ where i is odd.} \end{cases} \tag{5}$$

Alternatively, having defined a function step(t) as

$$\text{step}(t) = \begin{cases} 0 \text{ for } t < 0; \\ 1 \text{ otherwise,} \end{cases} \tag{6}$$

we may describe a normalized signal s(t) as:

$$s(t) = \sum_{i=0}^{2n-1} (-1)^i * \text{step}(t - t_i) \tag{7}$$

Observe that whatever the signal descriptions—Boolean algebra applies to normalized signals.

Let as label as **true** the value 1 of a normalized signal, and as **false** its value 0. Then, given two arbitrary normalized signals f(t) and g(t), possibly consisting of a different number of pulses of arbitrary timing, we can define standard Boolean operations as follows:

$$\textbf{not}\, f(t) = \text{step}(t) - f(t) \tag{8}$$

$$f(t)\,\textbf{and}\, g(t) = f(t) * g(t), \text{and finally} \tag{9}$$

$$f(t)\,\textbf{or}\, g(t) = f(t) + g(t) - f(t) * g(t) \tag{10}$$

These definitions allow us to formulate:

3.1 Self-test procedures for cochlear prostheses

Consider two arbitrary normalized signals f(t) and g(t), generated by two artificial hair cells of opposite orientation but of the same action potential and belonging to the same cochlear neighborhood. By *opposite orientation* we mean that both of them cannot be excitated simultaneously. For properly functioning such pair of artificial hair cells of a cochlear prosthesis the following conditions must hold for every t:

$$\begin{aligned} &f(t) \text{ and } g(t) = 0 \\ &f(t) \text{ and not } g(t) = f(t) \\ &g(t) \text{ and not } f(t) = g(t) \end{aligned} \tag{11}$$

This is so because f(t) and g(t) are mutually exclusive signals, while neither of them is the pure negation of another.

These test conditions can also be used to test cochlear prostheses as well as for hearing loss due to the loss of auditory cilia, caused by exposure to exceedingly high sound levels. Human hair cells have many cilia and initial hearing loss is usually not noticeable until large numbers of cilia are lost.

3.2 Audio location using pulse signals

Our simple methodology is sufficient for description of tasks like audio location.

Consider two hair cells with the same action potential, housed by two cochleae in two ears of an animal. A sound wave excites both cells, as per **Figure 6**.

An animal is capable of estimating the azimuth of the audio source by calculating the angle (shown) of the incoming sound. The essence of this well understood process is as follows: two hair cells, located in two cochleae of an animal are not excited simultaneously by an arriving sound wave. The delay in excitation of the hair cell more distant from the sound source can be used to calculate the extra distance the sound wave must travel to reach that cell (shown in **Figure 6**) Given that the base distance between the two cells (also shown in **Figure 6**) is an anatomical constant for

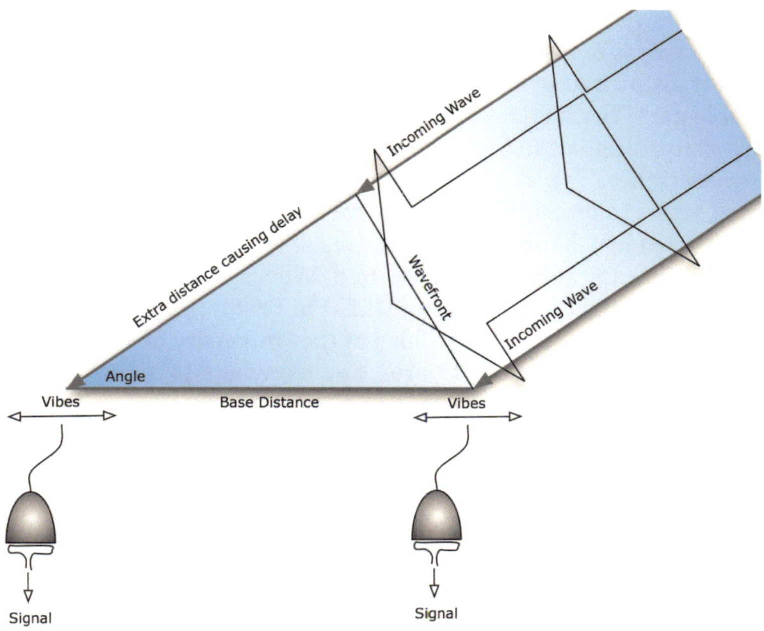

Figure 6.
Audio location process: One of two auditory cells in two different ears detects the same signal with a bit of delay.

a given animal, and the speed of sound in the medium the animal inhabits is also constant, then the angle of arrival of the sound wave can be calculated from the right triangle shown. In fact, an audio locating animal does not need to perform those complex trigonometric calculations. It just needs to turn its head to make both signals arrive simultaneously: it then faces in the direction of the incoming sound.

Observe further that for this method to work the length of the sound wave cannot be too long nor too short. Too long waves would not result in contrasting deflections of the corresponding cilia; for to short waves the uniqueness of the solution is lost (due to the periodic nature of the oscillations).

Optimal locating acuity occurs when the deflections of the cilia are of opposite phase. That is why the optimal sound wavelengths ensuring this remain in close correlation with the distance between two corresponding cells located within two ears of an animal. This explains why humans use frequencies much lower than bats, for example. It all has to do with different distances between ears of humans and bats. The square pulse nature of the signals generated by the hair cells enhances contrast between these signals, thus facilitating the audio location process.

The above examples are intended to demonstrate the capability of our approach to model processes already well understood. To gain understanding of more complex processes of audio pattern recognition, music, etc. we need to introduce several new concepts. We start with the design of the prosthetic device.

4. The cochlear model and prosthetic device

Our concept of a modular multi-channel device allows the number of supported channels to grow arbitrarily as technology advances. According to current practice, the device consists of two parts: the implantable part and the external part, worn by the patient. This is in order to maintain skin continuity thus avoiding infection. Both parts communicate via a trans-dermal electromagnetic link.

The external part is responsible for the formation of the multi-channel restorative signal and for transmission of the multiplexed signal via the electromagnetic link to the implantable part. The implantable part de-multiplexes the received signal and feeds proper channel signals to the relevant fibers of the cochlear nerve via a micro-array of tiny electrodes. The technological challenges of connecting microscopic multi-channel cables to proper fibers of a nerve are currently being addresses by work of several teams, led by Charles C. Della Santina at Johns Hopkins University (Vestibular Neuroengineering Lab), Daniel Merfeld, Wangsong Gong, and Richard Lewis at Massachusetts Eye and Ear Infirmary (MEEI) in Boston, James O. Phillips of the University of Washington, Andrei M. Shkel at the University of California, Irvine, Julius Georgiou at the University of Cyprus, and elsewhere [4]. Although these expert teams focus their work on the vestibular nerve, the technological challenges of connecting a micro-array of electrodes to any nerve remain the same.

In fact, we can use the cochlear nerve fiber layout to facilitate the connection. **Figure** 7 shows the cochlea and the outgoing nerve fibers. Observe that due to the spiral nature of the cochlea the central fibers of the nerve are connected to the cochlear tip and so are responsible for conveying information about low frequency components of the audio signal, while the outer fibers deal with high frequency components. Connection of a micro-array of electrodes to the nerve can therefore be a two-step procedure. First, we attach a micro-connector configured so that its center wires mate with center fibers, and then we fine-tune the connection by creating a

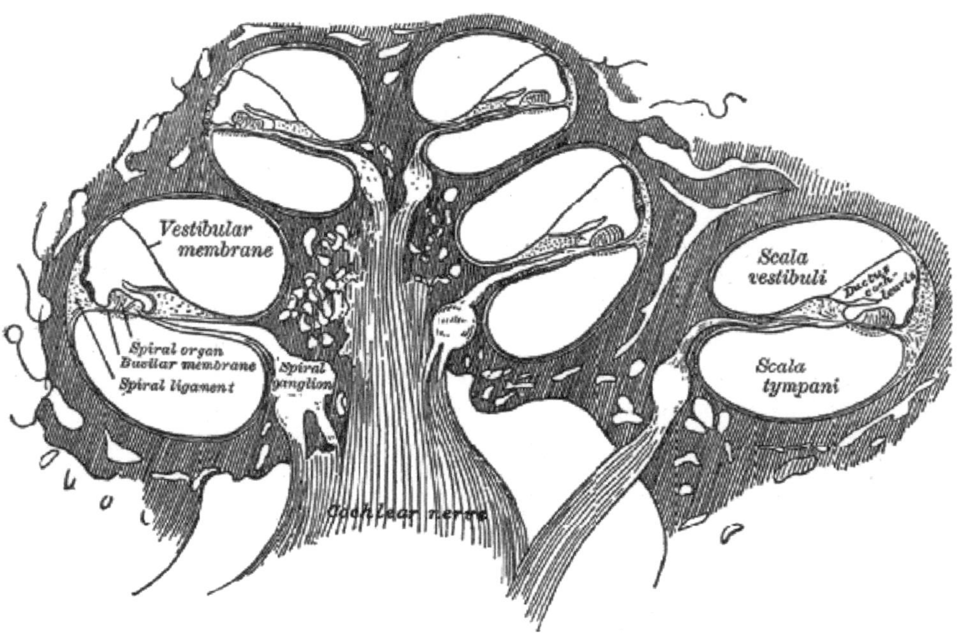

Figure 7.
Cochlear nerve layout: center fibers convey information regarding low frequency components of the audio signal; perimeter fibers deal with high frequencies.

detailed connection map, customized to each patient. We do that by passing stimulation signals to individual wires while asking the patient about frequencies perceived.

We focus now our attention on the formation of the restorative signal by an electronic device. That device consists of a microphone of a suitable directional characteristic, worn by the patient close to his non-functional ear, a transducer ensuring the transdermal connection, and a small electronic box, containing analog and digital circuitry.

To simulate our patient's cochlea, we will turn to the time-tested technology: that of a telegraph line. Early telegraph operators noticed that long telegraph lines tend to distort signals generated by telegraph keys. On the receiving end square pulse signals tended to have their edges rounded. When the line was too long, this distortion made the received signal unintelligible: dots of the Morse code would disappear, while dashes became dots with gentle slopes. To avoid this, telegraph lines have had certain maximum length, beyond which "repeaters" were used to refresh the signal. Early repeaters were just people transcribing the signals, later replaced by electrical devices.

While the goal of telegraph line builders was to maximize the quality of the signal and thus to maximize distance between repeaters by minimizing distortion, our goal is to minimize the size of the "bionic ear" worn by the patient. To that end we will construct a model of a bad telegraph line distorting the signal over short distances, and we will not use any repeaters.

A circuit shown in **Figure 8** is a model of a telegraph line segment or of neural axon segment. The wires of this segment present certain electrical resistance R [measured in ohms] and given that such line is never perfectly straight, a certain inductance L [henries]. The insulator between the two wires (air, plastic, etc.) is never perfect and so has a certain conductance G [siemens], and, together with the wires offers certain capacitance C [farads].

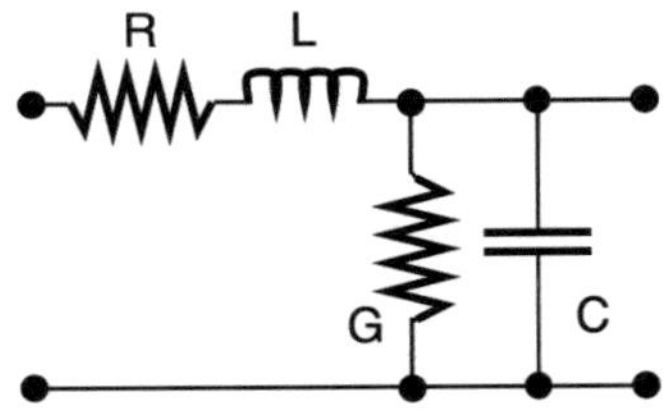

Figure 8.
Electrical model of a segment of a telegraph line or of a "bionic cochlea."

In physics the concepts of conductance G and resistance R are bound by an inverse relationship: G = 1/R. In the circuit of **Figure 8** the values of G and R are unrelated; they are just intrinsic parameters of a line segment.

Such circuit distorts an input signal applied to its left terminals by selectively attenuating harmonic components of the signal: higher harmonics are attenuated more than the lower harmonics. A telegraph line or our "bionic cochlea" nerve fiber can be represented by a finite sequence of such segments, as per **Figure 9**.

In a real cochlea information contained in higher harmonics of a signal is gathered close to the entry of the cochlea (i.e., close to the *oval window*), while only lower frequencies can penetrate to the end of the cochlea. The cochlea has a special terminator (called *round window*). That terminator has a dual role.

First, it allows the non-compressive endolymph, encased in a very hard bone, to move along the cochlea, thus agitating the auditory cilia. Indeed, in certain congenital abnormalities the round window may be missing or rigidly fixed. Not surprisingly, people so affected suffer a huge hearing loss of about 60 dB.

In a healthy cochlea, low frequency endolymph movements do not cause slowly moving liquid to exert sufficient drag on the cilia (it is analogous to the ease of moving a paddle through water sufficiently slowly). This translates to lowering of auditory sensitivity as frequency decreases, shown in **Figure 4**. On the other side of the audible frequency spectrum, high frequency waves are of small amplitude, and, attenuated further by the cilial inertia similarly fail to sufficiently deflect cilia, again resulting in loss of sensitivity as per **Figure 4**.

Second: The round window prevents sound waves from bouncing off the end of the cochlea and traveling back towards the oval window. Should this happen interference or even standing waves could form in the cochlea, resulting in humans hearing subjective sounds in absence of external stimuli (a condition known as *tinnitus*). A healthy cochlea is an echoless chamber.

Following those anatomical hints, we will sample signal in various points along our e-cochlea. This e-cochlea should be echoless, too. If it were infinitely long, it would certainly be echoless, as the signal could never reach its end to bounce back. This is impractical, though.

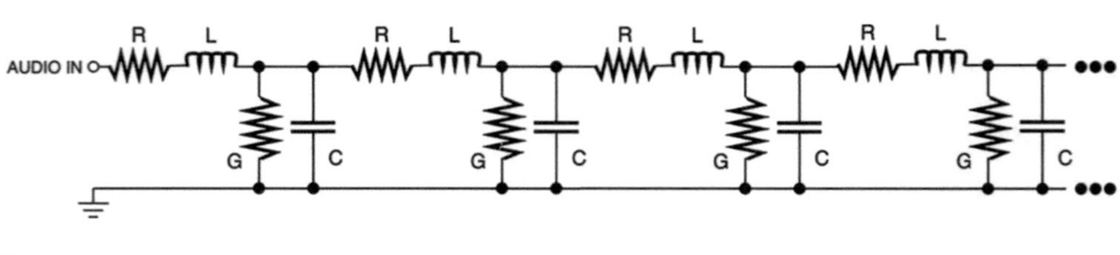

Figure 9.
Electrical model of a telegraph line or of a "bionic cochlea."

We can, however, calculate the input impedance of an infinitely long circuit depicted in **Figure 9**. Let that impedance be Z. If we terminate a finite circuit shown in **Figure 9** with a terminator Z (not shown), then viewed from the input side that circuit will be indistinguishable from an infinitely long circuit, and so will become echoless.

Incidentally, nature followed the same process when evolving cochleae. To increase audio acuity of more complex animals, it had to sample signals in many places along a cochlea, so the cochleae of higher animals had to become longer. In order then to fit them into a limited space of a cranial cavity in an extraordinarily hard bone the cochleae had to be coiled. Coiling a cochlea does not affect it acoustic properties much as coiling of a trumpet makes a trumpet smaller but does not affect its sound. With the exception of monotremes, all mammals have coiled cochleae.

We are now in a position to present the fundamental circuitry of our "bionic ear," as per **Figure 10**. The electric equivalent of an audio signal (for brevity called "audio signal" henceforth) is fed into an e-cochlea made of a large but finite number of segments, and properly terminated by an echoless terminator Z (not shown).

The input audio signal fed to each segment is also input to an analog sampling circuit equipped with a basic A/D converter. The output of this converter is **true** when its input voltage is positive and is **false** otherwise. In this way a pulsating digital signal is obtained. The A/D converter can be constructed from a single transistor oscillating between the cut-off and saturation states or a similar device. It simulates the axon hillock of an auditory neuron.

Given that on short time scales the audio signal is practically symmetric about the timeline, only the signal values exceeding certain positive reference voltages need be sampled. Every reference voltage is determined by the ratio of resistances R1/R2. When the voltage of the audio signal exceeds that threshold value, then the diode depicted in the diagram charges the capacitor Cx. As long as this capacitor is sufficiently charged, the A/D converter outputs the value **true**. The resistor Rx slowly discharges the capacitor Cx. A careful choice of the decay time constant RxCx, customizable to each patient, controls the minimum duration of each pulse. That time constant describes the dynamics of an auditory cell changing its electrochemical potential.

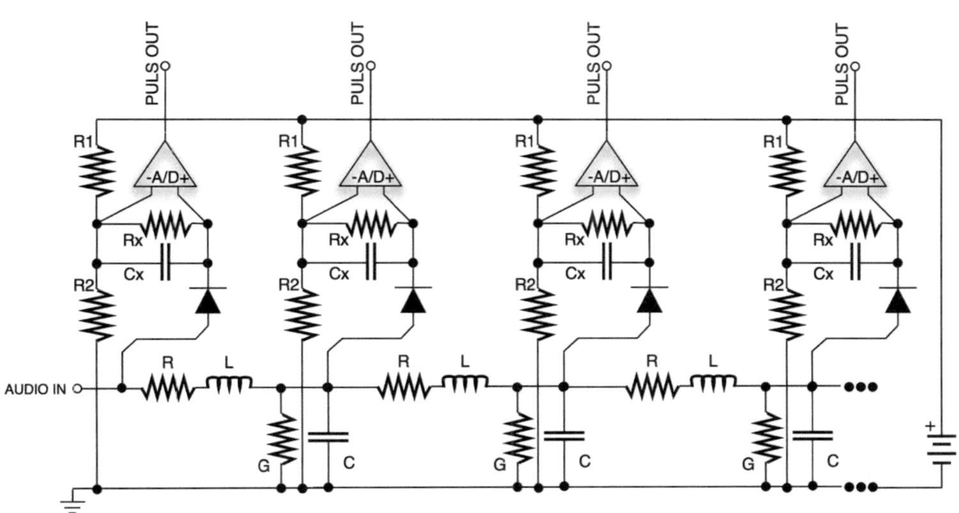

Figure 10.
Electrical model of a "bionic ear": each segment of the e-cochlea generates one digital signal.

Similarly, by adjusting values of the threshold ratio R1/R2 in each segment we can control the audio sensitivity of our e-cochlea to fit curves shown in **Figure 4**. Further tweaking is possible to customize this circuitry to the sensitivities and preferences of individual patients.

Note the simplicity of this design: Our "bionic ear" consists of a number of repeating segments, each segment yielding one channel of a digital signal. All segments are topologically identical, but may differ in element values R, L, G, and C to span the desired frequency spectrum in suitable number of steps, yielding the required number of channels. The last segment is capped with a suitable echoless terminator Z.

Due to current technological limitations this design probably does not allow us to create a sequence of 30,000 segments today, each segment generating a pulse signal to feed one fiber of the cochlear nerve, but it certainly overcomes current channel limitations. Furthermore, the modularity of the design allows us to build ever better, multi-channel bionic ears as technology improves.

This concludes our qualitative description of bionic ear electronics. To demonstrate that our device is capable of generating signals useful for sophisticated auditory perception, we need to introduce several mathematical concepts. We will also shed light on the way brain nuclei higher up the auditory pathway operate, with emphasis on audio pattern recognition and classification.

5. Variation on the theme of metric spaces

Mathematicians conceive a metric space as a set of objects, usually called "points," between which a way of measuring the distance has been defined. In everyday life we use Euclidean distance. However, this is only one of the many possible ways of measuring distances.

Let **S** be our space of interest.

Definition 1. Measure of distance: Any real-valued function d: $\mathbf{S} \times \mathbf{S} \rightarrow \mathbf{R}$ can be used as a measure of distance, provided that for all x, y, z $\in$ **S** it has the following properties:

$$d(x, x) = 0 \tag{12}$$

$$\text{if } x \neq y \text{ then } d(x, y) > 0,$$

$$\text{i.e.the distance between two distinct points cannot be zero;} \tag{13}$$

$$d(x, y) = d(y, x), \text{ i.e.the distance does not depend on the direction of measurement;} \tag{14}$$

$$d(x, z) \leq d(x, y) + d(y, z), \text{ i.e.the distance cannot be diminished by measuring it via some cleverly chosen intermediate point y.} \tag{15}$$

The last property is frequently called the *triangle law*, because the length of each side of a triangle cannot be greater than the sum of lengths of two other sides.

The properties (12) and (13) imply that the distance between any two points cannot be negative and is actually positive if the points are different. In fact, we can state.

Theorem 1: Given any real-valued function d: $\mathbf{S} \times \mathbf{S} \rightarrow \mathbf{R}$ suitable for measuring-distances between points in **S**, the equality d(x, y) = 0 for any x, y $\in$ **S** implies x = y.

Proof: The equality d(x, y) = 0 means that a shortest travel from x to y does not make us cover any distance, therefore x and y must coincide, that is, x = y. ■

As examples consider a two-dimensional space $\mathbf{R}^2$ and two points a = $\langle x_1, y_1 \rangle$ and b = $\langle x_2, y_2 \rangle$. We may define distance d(a, b) as:

$$\text{Euclidean distance}: d1(a, b) = \text{sqrt}\left((x_1 - x_2)^2 + (y_1 - y_2)^2\right) \quad \text{or} \tag{16}$$

$$\text{Manhattan distance}: d2(a, b) = |x_1 - x_2| + |y_1 - y_2| \quad \text{or} \tag{17}$$

$$\text{perhaps simply as}: d3(a, b) = \max\{|x_1 - x_2|, |y_1 - y_2|\} \tag{18}$$

All three functions d1, d2, and d3 meet the necessary requirements (12), (13), (14) and (15).

Definition 2. A metric space is the configuration $\langle \mathbf{S}, d \rangle$, where **S** is a set of points, and d is some measure of distance between them.

In our study we are frequently interested in measuring distance between subsets of **S**, rather than only between points of **S**. One of the simplest subsets of **S** is a *ball*.

Definition 3. A ball of radius r ≥ 0 around the point c ∈ **S** is the set

$$\{x \in \mathbf{S} | d(c, x) \le r\} \tag{19}$$

which we will denote as **B**(c, r) without mentioning either **S** or d when confusion can be avoided. The point c is called the center of the ball **B**.

Note: In older math textbooks the term "sphere" is frequently used instead of a "ball." This usage is currently being phased out, as we prefer now the "sphere" to mean the surface of a "ball."

Observe that the "shape" of a ball depends on the way we measure distance, as per **Figure 11**.

It is worth noticing that the "volumes" of such balls may depend on the metrics used. In particular, the Manhattan ball d2 is most specific about its center, that is, it has the smallest "volume" (i.e., area in $\mathbf{R}^2$), and also its metric function (17) computes faster than metrics (16) and (18). This is important for some of pattern recognition algorithms including visual and auditory perception, which, although fast and massively parallel, remain computationally intensive [2, 3].

A more detailed analysis of metric spaces can be found at [11].

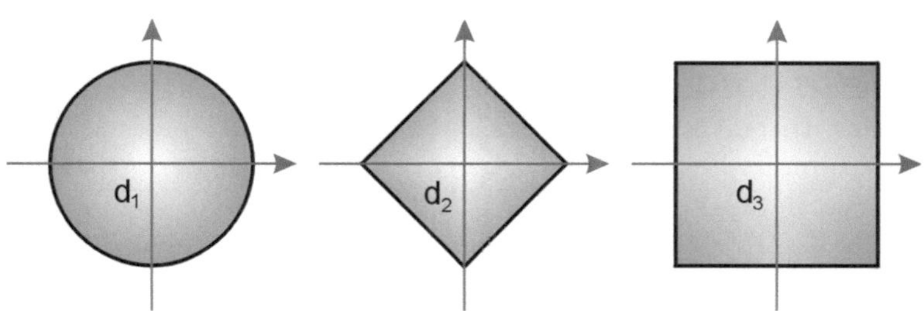

Figure 11.
The balls in $\mathbf{R}^2$ of same radius, with center in the origin of the system of coordinates, defined using metrics d_1, d_2, and d_3 in the previous example. Similar balls in $\mathbf{R}^3$ would be a sphere, an octahedron, and a cube, correspondingly. Generalizations of balls in higher-dimensional spaces are conceptually straightforward, although not easily drawn.

6. Computing distances between sets

Given any two non-empty sets **A**, **B** ⊂ **S** we need to construct a function D(**A**, **B**) to measure distance between **A** and **B**. That function should retain the properties (12), (13), (14) and (15). In particular, observe that the properties (12) and (13) imply that D(**A**, **B**) > 0 even if the sets **A**, **B** touch (i.e., have one common element), or intersect, or perhaps one of them contains another (**A** ⊂ **B** or **B** ⊂ **A**). In fact, we must construct function D such that D(**A**, **B**) = 0 if and only if **A** = **B**.

Let d be our chosen function for measuring distance between points of space **S**. We will use this function to construct our function D.

Definition 4. Distance between a point and a set: Let ⟨**S**, d⟩ be a metric space and let **A** ⊂ **S** be a non-empty set. A distance between a point x ∈ **S** and **A**, denoted δ (x, **A**) is given by

$$\delta(\mathrm{x}, \mathbf{A}) = \inf \{\mathrm{d}(\mathrm{x}, \mathrm{a}) | \mathrm{a} \in \mathbf{A}\} \tag{20}$$

It is the distance between x and a point a ∈ **A** closest to x. Using δ, let us define.

Definition 5. Pseudo-distance between two sets: Let ⟨**S**, d⟩ be a metric space and let **A**, **B** ⊂ **S** be two non-empty sets. A pseudo-distance from **A** to **B**, denoted Δ(**A**, **B**) is given by

$$\Delta(\mathbf{A}, \mathbf{B}) = \sup\{\delta(\mathrm{a}, \mathbf{B}) | \mathrm{a} \in \mathbf{A}\} \tag{21}$$

In other words, pseudo-distance from **A** and **B** is the distance from the most distant point a ∈ **A** to its closest point b ∈ **B**. It is not distance, but merely pseudo-distance, because it is unidirectional, that is, the property (14) does not hold, given that Δ(**A**, **B**) ≠ Δ(**B**, **A**) in general. To make it bidirectional, we define.

Definition 6. Distance between two sets: Let ⟨**S**, d⟩ be a metric space and let **A**, **B** ⊂ **S** be two non-empty sets. A distance between **A** and **B**, denoted D(**A**, **B**) is given by

$$\mathrm{D}(\mathbf{A}, \mathbf{B}) = \max \{\Delta(\mathbf{A}, \mathbf{B}), \Delta(\mathbf{B}, \mathbf{A})\} \tag{22}$$

We are ready now to demonstrate that our construction of D(**A**, **B**) has properties of a metric.

Theorem 2: Our newly constructed function D has the properties (12), (13), (14) and (15), and therefore can be used as a measure of distances between subsets of **S**.

Proof: Let ⟨**S**, d⟩ be a metric space and let **A**, **B**, **C** ⊂ **S** be non-empty sets. We have

1. **Property (12)** a.k.a. **reflexivity**: Let us compute D(**A**, **A**). Let us choose an arbitrary point a ∈ **A**. Using Definition 4 (see (20)) we obtain δ(a, **A**) = 0, because the closest target in **A** from a is a itself, as it belongs to **A**. From that it must follow that Δ(**A**, **A**) = 0 because the largest of all zeros is zero (peruse (21)). This implies further that D(**A**, **A**) = 0 because greater of two zeros is still a zero (see again (22)).

2. **Property (13):** Let **A** ≠ **B**. Both sets being not empty, we can find an a ∈ **A** such that a ∉ **B**, or b ∈ **B** such that b ∉ **A**, or both (if this were not the case, then the sets **A** and **B** would be equal). Given that at least one of a and b does not belong to both sets, we must have either δ(a, **B**) > 0 or δ(b, **A**) > 0 or both. From this we have either Δ(**A**, **B**) > 0 or Δ(**B**, **A**) > 0 or both, and so
D(**A**, **B**) > 0 as being greater of the previous two.

3. **Property (14)** a.k.a. **commutativity** follows directly from the Definition 6: D(**A**, **B**) = max {Δ(**A**, **B**), Δ(**B**, **A**)}, so the order of arguments does not matter when evaluating D(**A**, **B**).

4. **Property (15)** a.k.a. **triangle rule**: We need to show that D(**A**, **B**) ≤ D(**A**, **C**) + D(**C**, **B**).

A comment on travel from **A** to **B** via **C**: not any path will do. It is not sufficient to reach **C** from **A** at particular point $c_1 \in \mathbf{C}$ and then continue the trip from another point $c_2 \in \mathbf{C}$ to reach **B** to claim that we have traveled through **C**. Our itinerary must form a continuous path, that is, its first leg must end up at some point c ∈ **C** exactly where the second leg begins.

Let then the points a ∈ **A** and b ∈ **B** be arbitrarily chosen departure and destination points such that d(a, b) = D(**A**, **B**). Depending on the metric chosen the path from a to b of length d(a, b) may not be unique. However, each of such paths may or may not pass through our intermediate point c ∈ **C**. If it does, then we do not modify that path, and so its length does not change. If it does not, then we need to modify it to pass through c. In that situation the length of that path can only increase. Given that D(**A**, **B**) is computed using carefully chosen paths leading from a ∈ **A** to b ∈ **B** (or vice versa), such modifications of these paths can only result in leaving them intact or lengthening them, thus proving that D(**A**, **B**) ≤ D(**A**, **C**) + D(**C**, **B**). ■

Note that it also follows from this theorem that for our function D the Theorem 1 holds as well.

More importantly for the purposes of our chapter, observe that we may move the sets **A** and **B** within their space **S** so as to minimize D(**A**, **B**). Even then, for **A** and **B** being different, the residual value D(**A**, **B**) > 0 will remain.

With the information regarding the spatial positioning of sets **A** and **B** deliberately destroyed through such preprocessing, that residual value D(**A**, **B**) can be seen as measure of dissimilarity between sets. The function D can therefore serve also as a pattern classifier. With properly selected small value of ε > 0, the condition D(**A**, **B**) ≤ ε implies that **A** and **B** so preprocessed are sufficiently similar to be included in the same category.

7. Comparisons of audio patterns

We concern ourselves now with issues of pattern recognition, which in auditory domain call for comparison of audio signals. An audio signal is really a bundle of rectangular pulse signals traveling through fibers of a cochlear nerve. We will take full advantage of their properties arising from the fact that these elementary signals belong to time domain, that is, $\mathbf{R}^1$ space.

An audio pattern is an excerpt of an audio signal taken over a suitable time interval. Two audio patterns are similar, if all their elementary corresponding pulse signals are similar, that is, differ at most by an arbitrarily small time value of ε > 0.

7.1 Properties of elementary audio patterns

Our function D, although mathematically correct and theoretically useful in measuring distances and dissimilarities between sets, is only computable for sets belonging to $\mathbf{R}^1$ space (time domain). Readers interested in circumventing this limitation are directed elsewhere [2, 3].

Consider now two corresponding elementary signals, shown in **Figure 12**, as red and blue, for clarity. They are excerpted from two different signal bundles. Clearly, they are not identical. Are they then completely different and unrelated, or is one a subtle plagiarism on the theme of another? Without any numerical measure of their dissimilarity, any two experts may have three different opinions on this matter. We will use our function D as a reconciliation tool.

For the purposes of comparison two signal bundles must be aligned, that is, both must start at the same time, which we will denote as time zero. This means that in each signal bundle there is at least one elementary signal starting at time zero.

However, not all elementary signals in that bundle need to start simultaneously. Indeed, their relative timing is one of the intrinsic characteristics of each signal bundle. We can now define:

Definition 7: The dissimilarity between two signal bundles is the maximum dissimilarity between two corresponding elementary pulse signals in each signal bundle.

We therefore turn our attention to comparisons of elementary pulse signals.

Let us compare first signals consisting of one pulse each. **Figure 13** shows all possible relationships between such two signals. We will be calculating the value of $\Delta(\mathbf{A}, \mathbf{B})$, being the fundamental component of $D(\mathbf{A}, \mathbf{B})$. In other words, we will be measuring pseudo-distance from **A** to **B** (the pseudo-distance in the inverse direction is measured in identical way). For clarity, in our graphs **A** will be shown in red, **B** in blue.

Furthermore, we adopt the convention that the value t_{A0} and t_{A1} are the start and the stop times of pulse A, and the values t_{B0} and t_{B1} are accordingly the start and stop times of pulse B.

Translating the formula (21) into plain multi-disciplinary English we write:

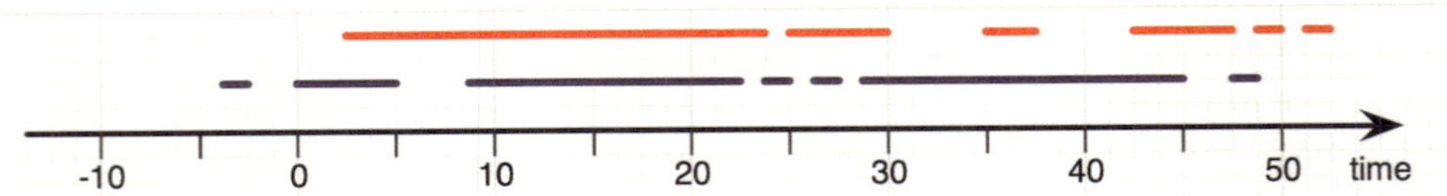

Figure 12.
Two pulse signals: are they really different? Unrelated? Or is there a similarity?

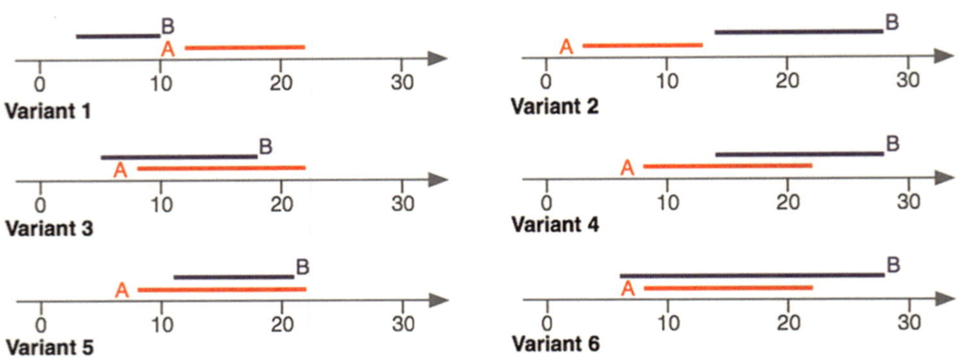

Figure 13.
Possible relationships between two pulse signals.

Pseudo-distance Δ (A, B) is the distance between the most distant point of A to its closest point in B.

This value describes the worst-case scenario when traveling from A to B in terms of the length of the shortest trip.

We are now in position to compute Δ(A, B) for all variants shown in **Figure 13**. We have:

$$\text{Variant } 1: \Delta(A,B) = |t_{A1} - t_{B1}|, \quad \text{Variant } 2: \Delta(A,B) = |t_{A0} - t_{B0}|,$$
$$\text{Variant } 3: \Delta(A,B) = |t_{A1} - t_{B1}|, \quad \text{Variant } 4: \Delta(A,B) = |t_{A0} - t_{B0}|,$$
$$\text{Variant } 5: \Delta(A,B) = \max\{|t_{A0} - t_{B0}|, |t_{A1} - t_{B1}\}, \text{Variant } 6: \Delta(A,B) = 0 \text{ because } A \subset B.$$

These variants can be easily identified and pseudo-distances computed, even by simple systems of several neurons. Observe symmetries in these expressions. On any parallel computer both values $| t_{A0} - t_{B0} |$ and $| t_{A1} - t_{B1} |$ can be calculated simultaneously, and then the proper value can be used as needed. Needless to say, we treat the brain as a parallel computer.

Do we have all the tools needed to compute distances between elementary pulse signals? Not yet. Not all elementary pulse signals consist of a single pulse each. In certain situations, two pulses in B may be needed to measure Δ(A, B). **Figure 14** depicts some of those cases. Signal A consists of one pulse as before, but signal B is now made out of two pulses. To cover these situations, we need to enhance our notation of pulse timing.

An elementary signal X consisting of n pulses we describe now as a tuple of 2n time values $< t_{X0,0}, t_{X0,1}, t_{X1,0}, t_{X1,1}, \ldots t_{Xn-1,0}, t_{Xn-1,1} >$. We number pulses in signal X starting at 0 and ending at n − 1. In that sense the notations $t_{X4,0}$ and $t_{X4,1}$ mean start and stop times of the fifth pulse of signal X (the fifth pulse has a number 4 because computer programmers like it that way!).

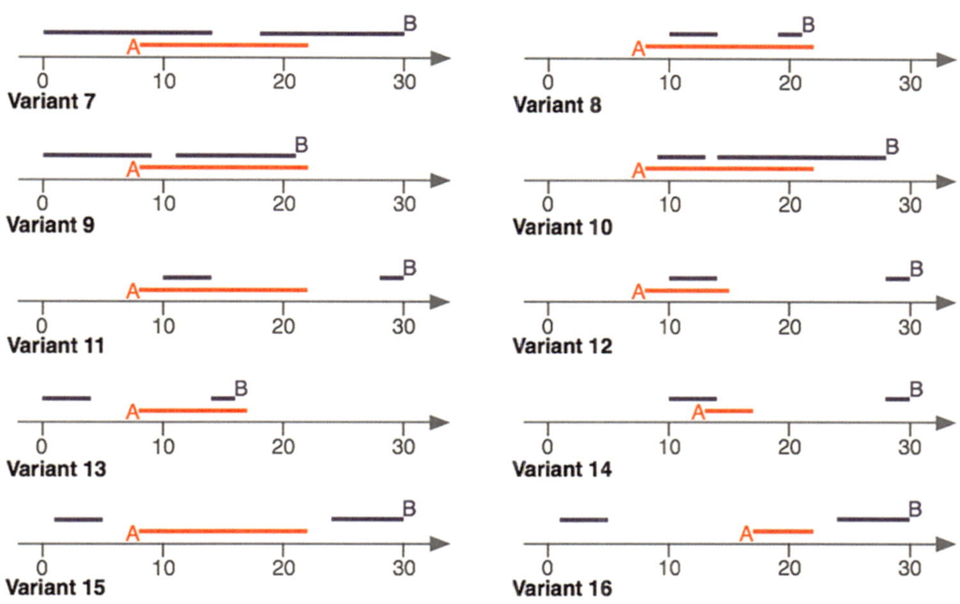

Figure 14.
Possible relationships between one-pulse signal A and two-pulse signal B.

Observe now what happens in variant 7 of **Figure 14**: the point in A most distant from B is that of timing in the middle of the gap between two pulses of B. We have here

$$\Delta(A, B) = |t_{B0,1} - t_{B1,0}|/2$$

More importantly, we have arrived at the following result:

Conclusion 1: When measuring pseudo-distances Δ(A, B) the points in A (if any) that are in the middle of gaps in B (if any) must also be considered, as well as the start and end points of A. Still, only the end points in B are of interest.

Therefore, in variant 8 the value Δ(A, B) must be calculated as

$$\Delta(A, B) = \max \{|\, t_{A0,0} - t_{B0,0}|, |t_{B0,1} - t_{B1,0}|/2, |t_{A0,1} - t_{B1,1}|\}$$

Consider now the difference between variants 11 and 12. In variant 11 the pulse A extends beyond the middle of the gap between pulses in B, while in variant 12 it does not. Therefore, when calculating Δ(A, B) for variant 11, the value of the expression $| tB_{0,1} - tB_{1,0} |/2$ must be considered, while in variant 12 the existence of the second pulse can be ignored when calculating Δ(A, B) (although it is still relevant for calculation Δ(B, A)). Indeed, should there be more pulses in B following the second pulse of B (variant 12), they all could be ignored when calculating Δ(A, B). Similar situation can arise when a multi-pulse signal B is timed so that the leading pulses of B can be ignored. This is good news, as this situation leads to vastly simplified neural calculations. Simplicity bestows speed; for survival speed is of essence!

Note further that the calculated values of Δ(A, B) depend on whether or not they are arrived at in real time. As an example, consider the situation depicted in variant 13 shown in **Figure 14**. According to our analysis, the pseudo-distance Δ(A, B) value is $\Delta(A, B) = |tB_{0,1} - tB_{1,0}|/2$. This is established knowing *a priori* that signal B consists of two pulses. If, however, we do the comparison between A and B in real time and current time is 12 units, then we are in the situation where the first pulse of B already ended but the second pulse did not begin. We cannot even know whether the second pulse exists. We have no choice but to keep calculating the distance between that part of A which we have experienced already and the only part of the pulse of B we heard so far. This will overestimate the value of Δ(A, B). That value will drop off immediately when we hear the onset of the second pulse of B. In fact, we have established now the following:

Conclusion 2: The calculated values of Δ(A, B) are a function of time. This function is continuous when we have an *a priori* knowledge of all pulses in A and B (i.e., we compare patterns A and B previously stored in memory), but only piecewise continuous if we calculate Δ(A, B) in real-time (i.e., without such *a priori* knowledge).

In short: When computing Δ(A, B) in real time, the number of pulses of B to consider is further limited. Only the pulses experienced so far can be considered. This simplification further enhances the speed of calculation thus increasing our chances of survival. The fact that our calculation is less exact is immaterial; our foe suffers from the same handicap.

If we survive the encounter with our foe, when safe we can replay both patterns from memory, refining our calculation and survival strategy. When at leisure we have more time to safely indulge in more complex calculations, refining our forecasting models.

This also explains why we enjoy the same recording of music differently depending on whether we hear it for the first time or not.

A question then arises: Suppose we enjoy a piece of music we hear for the first time. If that pleasure is tied to a certain comparison process, what are we comparing that piece to?

Conclusion 3: When listening to a piece of music (even for the first time) we keep predicting its future passages, on the basis of most recent passages in a certain active time interval. In that sense music must adhere to a certain "grammar" to be found pleasurable.

We are now ready to create a formalism of comparison of two elementary pulse signals.

7.2 Comparisons of elementary audio patterns

Given two multi-pulse elementary patterns A and B, we need to calculate their dissimilarity as a distance D(A, B) = max {Δ(A, B), Δ(B, A)} as per formula (22). Again, we focus our attention at calculating the value Δ(A, B) (The value Δ(B, A) is computed in the same way).

Let A consist of n pulses, while B consists of m pulses. We can represent A and B as follows:

$$A = \bigcup_{i=0}^{n-1} A_i \quad \text{and} \quad B = \bigcup_{j=0}^{m-1} B_j \tag{23}$$

where A_i and B_j are single pulses.

The value of Δ(A, B) can now be calculated as:

$$\Delta(A, B) = \max \{\Delta(A_i, B) | i = 0..n\} \tag{24}$$

In fact, we can accelerate this computation. We have already observed that when calculating Δ(A, B), not all pulses of B are of interest as possible closest destinations on our travel from A_i to B. We can calculate Δ(A, B) more efficiently as

$$D(A, B) = \max \{\Delta(A_i, B^*) | i = 0..n\} \tag{25}$$

where B* is a subset of consecutive pulses of B, namely

$$B^* = \bigcup_{j=k(i)}^{l(i)} B_j \tag{26}$$

where k(i) and l(i) are the first and last pulses of this consecutive sub-sequence of interest when calculating the pseudo-distance from Ai to B.

To give formal justification to this computational short-cut, we need to establish the following:

Theorem 3: Let A and B be two multi-pulse elementary patterns defined as per (23). When calculating the values of Δ(Ai, B), not all pulses of B are relevant. We can limit our attention to a subset of consecutive pulses of B, namely

$$B^* = \bigcup_{j=k(i)}^{l(i)} B_j$$

where k, which depends on i is an index of the first pulse of interest, and l, which also depends on i, is an index of the last pulse of interest.

Proof: Consider an arbitrarily chosen single pulse $A_i \subseteq A$. The starting moment of this pulse, timed at $t_{Ai,0}$ may or may not coincide with a pulse of B. If it does, then that pulse of B is the first pulse of interest. We call it B_k. The pulses preceding B_k (if any) cannot be the target destinations on our journey from A_i to B, because at the moment $t_{Ai,0}$ we are already in B.

If it does not, then the most recent pulse of B preceding the moment $t_{Ai,0}$ is our first pulse of interest. Again, we call it B_k. As before, the pulses preceding B_k (if any) cannot be the target destinations on our journey from A_i to B, because the trip from A_i to B_k is shorter.

In a special case that there is no pulse of B preceding the moment $t_{Ai,0}$ the first pulse of B is B_k.

To identify the last pulse of interest B_l we proceed similarly. The ending moment of pulse A_i, timed at $t_{Ai,1}$ may or may not coincide with a pulse of B.

If it does, then that pulse of B is the last pulse of interest. We call it B_l. The pulses following B_l (if any) cannot be the target destinations on our journey from A_i to B, because at the moment $t_{Ai,1}$ we are already in B.

If it does not, then the most imminent pulse of B following the moment $t_{Ai,1}$ is our last pulse of interest. Again, we call it B_l. As before, the pulses following B_l (if any) cannot be the target destinations on our journey from A_i to B, because the trip from A_i to B_l is shorter.

In a special case that there is no pulse of B following the moment $t_{Ai,1}$ the last pulse of B is B_l. ■

In plain multi-disciplinary English, all this means: it is possible to compare two elementary pulse signals by scanning them simultaneously and chronologically, even in real time. In this situation each signal we need to place in a moving time window, containing relevant pulses only, and keep advancing that window as time goes on.

As said before, every audio signal is a bundle of elementary signals, and therefore comparison of two audio signals also involves usage two advancing time windows. This is not new: we do that intuitively all the time when listening to music. We keep certain passages in a moving time window (i.e., some form of active memory). We consider these passages "current" and give them special attention. We feel pleasure if they continue to remain within a certain anticipated "grammar." Older passages are kept in another, longer term memory.

We have been listening to and enjoying music since time immemorial. Until now it was just a beautiful emotion. Now we have a mathematical model of that emotion.

8. Final thoughts and recommendations

We are well on our way in gaining insight how our brains work. They are pattern comparison machines. When comparing complex patterns (visual, auditory, gustatory, etc.) complex patterns are decomposed into arrays of simper patterns on which the comparisons can easily be made. These simple comparisons are made in real time and their results are then consolidated into a general conclusion about the complex patterns.

Our analysis of audio signal comparison processes makes us further deduce that:

- Two audio signal bundles must consist of the same number of elementary pulse signals to be comparable, and these elementary signals must be compared pairwise;

- When an elementary signal in one bundle ceases to exist (due to an accident or a disease), the corresponding pulse signal in another bundle is not fully useful to the brain;

- Implanting two incompatible cochlear prostheses in one patient is a grave error in the art, as they generate incompatible thus incomparable bundle signals;

- Implanting only one prosthesis is therefore an equally grave blunder, unless it is fully compatible with a healthy cochlea;

- Cochlear prostheses should therefore be implanted in pairs and tuned simultaneously to each patient. Such tuning should be an inherent part of the implantation procedure.

In the audio domain two patterns consisting of a different number of elementary patterns cannot be similar—they are intrinsically of a different kind. They cannot be readily compared. Children frequently ask a vexing question: "Daddy, when both of us listen to a piece of music we like, do we feel exactly the same sense of pleasure?" The correct answer is: these feelings are subjective, unknowable to others; they arise in our brains as responses to our individual audio signals. It has been said that each human has approx. 30,000 fibers in the cochlear nerve, but the actual numbers vary among the individuals. Also vary the numbers of cilia, geometries of cochleae, ossicles, etc. No two individuals are alike, and their audio signals are mutually incompatible. So are their emerging feelings of pleasure.

No wonder that the challenges in constructing cochlear prostheses are daunting! No single cochlear prosthesis will fit everybody. It must be customized to an individual.

In the current practice things are done the other way around. Every implant manufacturer swears that his device is "best" but dares to implant it into selected patients only, counting on the plasticity of their brains to adapt to the device. To makes things worse, we tend to implant only one device per person—to avoid "complications." What complications? In fact, we introduce here unnecessary complications—humans (and other animals) have evolved to have two very similar ears. To ask of the human brain to adapt within a single lifespan to two different and mutually incompatible "ears," thus generating signals not readily comparable is to ask too much! Practical problems emerge, viz.: how to perform audio location if you have two different hearing organs generating incompatible signals? No wonder that the current implant success rate leaves much to be desired.

Our approach offers new promises, but first and foremost we should customize the cochlear prostheses to our patients, not the other way around. We are well on our way.

Illustration credits

Figure 1. Chittka L. Brockmann: Anatomy of the human ear. Wikimedia Commons. Available from: http://en.wikipedia.org/wiki/File:Anatomy_of_the_Huma n_Ear.svg [Accessed: 13 June 2010], Creative Commons Attribution 2.5 GenericLicense.

Figure 2. Cochlear cross-section. Wikimedia Commons. Available from: http:// en.wikipedia.org/wiki/File:Cochlea-crosssection.svg [Accessed: 13 June 2010], GNU Free Documentation license v. 1.2.

Figure 4. Contours of equal loudness. ISO 226:2003 revision.
Figure 7. Layout of the cochlear nerve. Wikipedia. Available from: http://upload.wikimedia.org/wikipedia/commons/b/bc/Gray928.png [Accessed: 17 July 2010], Public domain.

Acknowledgements

The author would like to thank his brother, Dr. W. Gregory Wojcik, MD, for his patient verbal advice and consultations on matters of biology and anatomy.

Author details

Wlodzimierz ("Vlad") Wojcik
Department of Computer Science, Brock University, St. Catharines, Ontario, Canada

*Address all correspondence to: vwojcik@brocku.ca

References

[1] Shannon RV, Zeng FG, Wygonski J, Kamath V, Ekelid M. Acoustic simulations of cochlear implants. Available from: http://www.healthaffairs.uci.edu/hesp/Simulations/simulationsmain.htm [Accessed: September 2010]

[2] Wojcik V, Comte P. Algorithms for speedy visual recognition and classification of patterns formed on rectangular imaging sensors. Neurocomputing. 2010;**74**(1–3): 140-154. DOI: 10.1016/j.neucom.2009.10.029

[3] Wojcik V, Comte P. Algorithms for speedy visual recognition and classification of patterns formed on rectangular imaging sensors. Technical Report: #CS-08-07. Department of Computer Science, Brock University. Available from: http://www.cosc.brocku.ca/files/downloads/research/cs0807.pdf [Accessed: July 2007]

[4] Della Santina CC. Regaining balance with bionic ears. Scientific American. [Accessed: April 2010]

[5] Crawford J. Living without a balancing mechanism. British Journal of Ophthalmology. 1964;**48**(7):357-360

[6] Minor LB. Gentamicin-induced bilateral vestibular hypofunction. Journal of the American Medical Association. 1998;**279**(7):541-544

[7] Della Santina CC et al. A multichannel semicircular canal neural prosthesis using electrical stimulation to restore 3-D vestibular sensation. IEEE Transactions on Biomedical Engineering. 2007;**54**(6):1016-1030

[8] Standring S et al. Gray's Anatomy: The Anatomical Basis of Clinical Practice. 40th ed. New York, NY: Elsevier; 2009

[9] Shannon-Hartley Theorem. Wikipedia. Available from: http://en.wikipedia.org/wiki/Shannon-Hartley_theorem [Accessed: September 2010]

[10] Gokhale AA. Introduction to Telecommunications. 2nd ed. Florence, KY: Thomson Delmar Learning; 2004

[11] Gleason AM. Elements of Abstract Analysis. Boston: Jones and Bartlett Publishers; 1991

Chapter 9

Hearing Restoration through Optical Wireless Cochlear Implants

Stylianos E. Trevlakis,
Alexandros-Apostolos A. Boulogeorgos and
George K. Karagiannidis

Abstract

In this chapter, we present two novel optical wireless-based cochlear implant architectures: (i) optical wireless cochlear implant (OWCI) and (ii) all-optical cochlear implant (AOCI). Both the architectures aim to decisively improve the reliability and energy efficiency of hearing restoration devices. To provide design and development guidelines, we document their main components, discuss the particularities of the transdermal optical channel, and provide the analytical framework for their accurate modeling. Building upon this framework, we extract closed-form formulas that quantify the communication, the stimulation, and the overall performance. An overall comparison of OWCI and AOCI, as well as conventional cochlear implants, accompanied by future research directions summarizes this chapter. Our findings reveal that both the OWCI and the AOCI outperform conventional cochlear implant approaches; thus, they are identified as promising architectures for the next generation of cochlear implants.

Keywords: all-optical cochlear implants, biomedical applications, cell stimulation, neural stimulation, optical wireless cochlear implants, optical wireless communications, optogenetics

1. Introduction

The healthy ear functions much like a receiver (Rx) of acoustic signals, which can be described as time-varying pressure waves in a specific frequency range (20–20,000 Hz). These signals propagate toward the cochlear, which analyzes them based on their spectral content. Specifically, each pressure wave traveling inside the cochlea not only actuates inner and outer hair cells at different locations along its length based on the frequency components of the wave, but also determines the intensity of the perceived sound according to the amplitude of the wave [1]. The various spiking characteristics of the spiral ganglion neurons, such as spike rate, number, and location, encode the amplitude and frequency of the sound.

The most common sensory defect is hearing loss, which plagues more than 466 million people around the world and is mostly caused by cochlear abnormalities [2]. When unaddressed, hearing loss can negatively impact the quality of life in various ways, such as social isolation, limited education, and unemployment, which are estimated to cost 980 billion dollars annually. To counterbalance this, substantial research effort has been directed toward neuron regenerative techniques, such as pharmacological, gene, as well as cell therapies [3, 4]. Unfortunately, none of the aforementioned approaches is considered to be close to clinical use. Therefore, the most successful hearing restoration approaches to this day are based on cochlear implants (CIs). Of note, CIs can be used in almost all forms of hearing loss.

Conventional CIs are comprised of two parts: one external and one implanted. The former houses a sound receiver and the processor, while the latter contains the stimulation unit. Specifically, the captured sound signal is decomposed to its major frequency components that are assigned to the corresponding channels of the stimulation unit. Each channel delivers the electrical stimulation signal to the spiral ganglion neurons that match the frequency content of the decomposed electrically encoded sound signal. However, due to the relatively high electrical conductivity of the cochlea, the applied electrical stimulation spreads to nearby spiral ganglion neurons, thus stimulating wider spectral windows than the appropriate one. In conjunction with their low-dynamic range [5], conventional CIs offer limited spectral and intensity sound encoding, which is proven to be detrimental for their hearing restoration capabilities [6].

In this chapter, we introduce the major advances that paved the way for the revolution of CIs and the realization of hearing restoration. Initially, we investigate the current state of the art of hearing restoration through CIs. Next, an in-depth analysis of most promising techniques of light-based hearing restoration is presented. Finally, we offer design guidelines as well as future directions for the next generation of CIs.

2. Background

To aid the reader in understanding the requirements of hearing restoration, we provide some background that covers the CIs' evolution since their conceptualization as well as the current research progresses toward the next generation of CIs (**Figure 1**).

2.1 Evolution of CIs

The concept of hearing restoration through the electrical stimulation of the auditory nerve was conceived by André Djourno and Charles Eyriés in 1957. In their attempt to restore the functionality of the facial nerve through electrical signal applied via a wire, the deaf patient experienced auditory sensations [7]. Based on these findings, multiple attempts were made around the world to develop the first CI with William House performing the first implantation in 1972 [8, 9]. Moreover, the first cochlear implant manufacturing company was founded in 1982 under the name MedEl Corporation, closely followed by Cochlear Limited in 1984, and Advanced Bionics in 1996.

Since their creation, CI companies have iteratively updated their architecture designs, hardware, and optimizing stimulation techniques. The first generation of CIs was released in the early 1980s and included Nucleus 22 and Comfort CI, combined analog signal processing strategies with a multichannel stimulation unit that housed 22 and 4 channels, respectively. These designs were followed by the initial model of Advanced Bionics called Clarion in 1996 that was encased in a ceramic case, contained

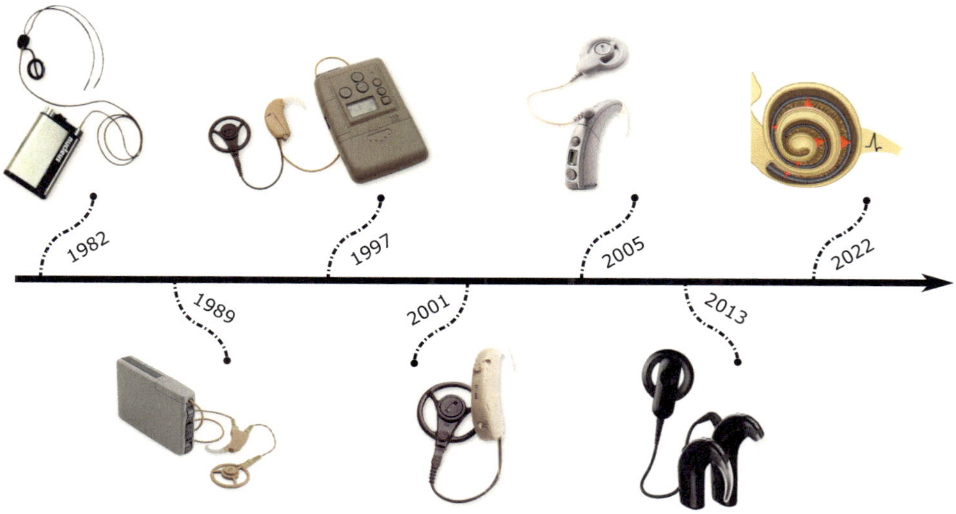

Figure 1.
The evolution of CIs from 1982, when the first CI manufacturing company was founded, until the current state-of-the-art research that validated the feasibility of optogenetics-enabled optical CIs.

eight channels, and used rechargeable batteries. The second generation included Clarion II, Nucleus 24 Contour, and Combi 40+. These were introduced in the market with 24 electrodes and new sound processors with novel features such as precurved electrode arrays, backward compatibility, frequency modulation capabilities, dual electrodes, and behind-the-ear external components. However, in the early 2000s, completely redesigned highly customizable CI models, namely, Freedom, Pulsar, and HiRes90k, were developed. Their modularity and customization options were the distinguishing factors for these new models that were available in straight or precurved, standard, medium, condensed, and split electrode array architectures, based on the individual particularities of the cochlea of each patient. Moreover, these electrodes were encased in flexible plastic and housed a plastic tip that enabled nontraumatic implantation. In the era after 2010, the latest iterations of CIs have been focused toward higher fidelity sound that enhances the perception of music through state-of-the-art sound processing, wireless control, and software-enabled programability, as well as waterproof designs.

2.2 What the next-generation CI should be?

The utilization of light-based communications and stimulation has been proposed as a promising alternative for electrical hearing restoration techniques. The superior communication performance of optical wireless communications in trandermal applications revealed the benefits that can be achieved by utilizing light for the communication between the external and implanted components of CIs [10, 11]. Moreover, optogenetics was initially reported by Izzo et al. [12] and has been proven achieve more efficient coding of the spectral information of sound due to its higher temporal confinement compared to the electronic stimulation techniques [13–15]. Although optical stimulation has great potential, it exhibits increased energy requirements for achieving the actuation of spiral ganglion neurons, and thus, future research is necessary for developing more energy-efficient techniques [16]. Finally, the combination of optogenetics and optical wireless communications offers great promise for the realization of an all-optical CI architecture capable of achieving unprecedented performance [17].

3. Current research progress

Two main research directions remain to be investigated. First, transdermal communication plays an important role in propagating the sound information captured by the microphone of the external component toward the one implanted. Conventional CIs are based on magnetic coupling, a near-field technique that uses low radio frequencies (RFs) in the range of 5–50 MHz for communication [18, 19]. The required power of conventional CIs lies around some decades milliwatts. Although this technology has been successfully applied in the majority of CIs, it suffers from low data rates, which constrain the performance of artificial hearing aids in their attempt to simulate high-quality normal hearing [20–22]. In addition, the aforementioned spectral window is used by numerous applications, which generate a great amount of interference that diminishes the quality of communication [23–25]. On the other hand, the optical activation of the auditory nerve via optogenetics has been experimentally verified, but the propagation of the spiral ganglion neuron potential through the auditory pathway toward the brain and its successful perception have yet to be demonstrated [26]. Moreover, the superiority of optical over electrical cell stimulation must be validated in order to justify the research effort toward the all-optical cochlear implant (AOCI) [17]. Recently, multiple experiments have progressed these goals by implanting novel tiny optical fibers in animals models of human sensorineural hearing loss [27–29].

3.1 Communications

To overcome the aforementioned CI restrictions, researchers have investigated the viability of transdermal wireless networks that operate in nonstandard frequencies. Owing to increased bandwidth, surprisingly high tolerance to external interference, and partial skin transparency at near-infrared wavelengths, optical wireless communications have been applied to transdermal channels instead of the traditional RF-based techniques [30, 31]. In the past decade, numerous contributions have experimentally verified the practicality of transdermal optical links [32–36]. Abita established a transdermal optical link from the inside toward the outside component of a medial system achieving high-data-rate communications [32], while Ackermann et al. investigated the design principles and tradeoffs that are entangled to optical-based CIs [33, 37]. Moreover, Liu introduced a high-data-rate transdermal optical link for implantable biomedical systems with high energy efficiency under the assumption of deterministic misalignment [24]. Similarly, the interactions between data rate, transmission power, receiver characteristics, and tissue thickness as well as their impact on the system's performance were evaluated for transdermal optical links applied in neural signal extraction scenarios [38]. In addition, the same authors validated the proposed system by conducting *in vivo* experiments that achieved 2×10^{-7} bit error rate (BER) and 100-Mbps data rate under stochastic misalignment, but with relatively high power consumption in the order of 2 mW [36]. On the contrary, a novel retroflective architecture was presented for transdermal optical links [34], while Liu proposed a bidirectional transdermal optical link [35].

Building upon the aforementioned contributions, the development of optical-based CIs needs to leverage breakthrough technologies while taking into consideration the particularities of the transdermal and in-body optical channels, the space and energy design limitations, as well as the directionality of the optical links. Moreover, a novel information-theoretic framework is required for the design of energy-efficient physical and medium access schemes, as well as the development of simultaneous light information and power transfer policies and resource allocation strategies. Motivated by the above, recent research effort has been devoted toward delivering safety and high quality of experience in CIs and identifying the critical technology gaps and the appropriate enablers.

3.2 Neural stimulation

After communicating the information from the external environment toward the implanted component of the CI, the techniques of neural stimulation must be applied in order to excite the cochlear spiral ganglion neurons, which, in turn, will generate the desire action potential that will propagate along the acoustic nerve toward the brain. Over the years, various methods of neural stimulation have been developed. These can be categorized based on the nature of the applied stimulus as acoustic, thermal, magnetic, chemical, optical, and electrical, with the last ones being the most recognized [39]. Specifically, electrical neural stimulation is the most common technique and has been used in a wide gamut of biomedical applications [40–42]. Electrical neural stimulation applies an electrical stimulus (voltage, current [40], or charge [42]) on the target nerves that manipulates their membrane potential so that it exceeds a certain threshold and, therefore, generates or inhibits action potentials. Specifically, deep brain and cardiac muscle stimulation techniques that use voltage control mechanisms have been investigated with regard to power consumption [41, 43], while current-controlled electrical neural stimulation in CIs is characterized by power waste in the tissue that leads to limited longevity and tissue damage [40]. Voltage-controlled electrical neural stimulation is proven to be more power efficient and less complex, but with very limited stimulus tuning options that result in faster degradation of the electrode contacts. The opposite is valid for current-controlled electrical neural stimulation that can apply fine-tuned charge to the electrodes but exhibits lower power efficiency. Finally, charge control mechanisms for electrical neural stimulation have been applied on the peripheral neural system [42] and offer a middle ground between stimulus control and power consumption. Despite the control mechanism, the determining factors of electrical neural stimulation techniques include human safety, energy efficiency, stimulation waveform, and spatial resolution. The latter significantly affects the stimulation accuracy and is correlated with the distance from the targeted neurons as well as the size of the electrode, which is limited by maximum permissible charge per tissue surface and the electrode's manufacturing process. In addition, the unique characteristics of different types of neurons greatly affect their response to stimulations with variable waveform properties, such as amplitude, width, and frequency. To this end, a great amount of research effort has been devoted toward optimizing the waveform for the stimulus [44–47]. Finally, throughout the optimization procedure of electrical neural stimulation techniques, safety for humans must be ensured.

The solution to the several limitations of electrical neural stimulation was introduced almost two decades ago in the form of optical neural stimulation that uses light for the actuation and control of neurons. Specifically, light-gated ion channels found in proteins, termed opsins, have been proven to mediate light-driven action potentials in mammalian neurons by manipulating the polarization of their membrane and, therefore, suppressing or exciting them. Optical neural stimulation is highly dependent on the type of the utilized opsin, which incentivized research toward experimentally verifying its performance in terms of precision, accuracy, frequency, and scalability [48–51]. Optical neural stimulation was successfully applied in the motor control system of rodents [48], while the causal relationship of frequency-based optical neural stimulation and behavior state transitions was verified [49]. The increased specificity of exciting neurons was illustrated through efficiently mapping the spatial distribution of synaptic inputs [50]. Moreover, a high-precision optical neural stimulation technique for inhibiting neurons with temporal fidelity was developed [51]. The performance of this technique was evaluated based on novel key performance indicators such as light sensitivity. The aforementioned works illustrate that the development of opsins offering stable performance over multiple stimulations is accompanied by long desensitization periods and short channel-off durations. To this end, research was intensified toward developing opsins with different kinetic features and wavelength sensitivity for monitoring and controlling biological processes in subcellular and cellular levels [52, 53]. A major breakthrough was achieved with the application of channelrhodopsin 2 (ChR2) in mammalian neurons that enabled accurate stimulation with light pulses [54]. Since its development, ChR2 has been heavily investigated, and multiple variants have been introduced with applications in cardiology [55–58] and neuroscience [59, 60]. The performance of these variants greatly outperforms electrical neural stimulation in terms of stimulation pulse intensity and frequency (up to 200 Hz), as well as the ability to trigger large current action potentials with higher fidelity [61, 62].

4. Light-based hearing restoration

Based on the literature review presented in the previous section, the main bottlenecks of CIs are low accuracy and low precision of nerve stimulation methods, bandwidth scarcity and constraint capacity of RF communication techniques, and high energy consumption of both. To this end, we present two architectures capable of mitigating the effect of these limitations and even eliminating them [11, 17].

4.1 Optical wireless cochlear implant

The utilization of optical wireless communications in order to develop CI transdermal optical links has been recently investigated [11], where the authors proposed a novel system architecture, termed optical wireless cochlear implant (OWCI), that improves the power and spectral efficiency as well as the reliability of the transdermal optical link. Moreover, in the same contribution [11], the capabilities and feasibility of the OWCI are evaluated and design guidelines are provided. The main comparison points between OWCIs and conventional CIs are illustrated in **Table 1**. In addition, the presented advances in the communications of CIs are in line with optical neural stimulation advances on the acoustic nerve [21, 63–67].

The unique technical contributions of the OWCI entail the establishment of a novel system model for transdermal optical links that incorporates the various design variables such as the stochastic misalignment between the receiver (RX) and the transmitter (TX), the scale of the optical components, the skin thickness, and the

OWCIs	Conventional CIs
Increased data rate	Low data rate
Abundant bandwidth	Limited bandwidth
High power efficiency	Low power efficiency
Safer for the human body	Questionable safety
Mature technology with promise of	Mature technology
higher performance in the same scale	with compact designs
Low solar and ambient light interference	Very high electronic interference
Stringent alignment requirements	**Susceptible misalignment**
Multiple design guidelines	**Mature standardization**
(IrDA, EU COST 1101, IEC LSS, IEEE Std 1073.3.2-2000, etc.)	**(IEEE Std 1073.3.2-2000, IEEE 802.15.4, etc.)**

Table 1.
OWCIs versus conventional CIs (bold fonts demonstrate the advantages).

transmission power. The external component of the OWCI is comprised of a microphone, the TX, and a digital signal processing (DSP) unit, while the implanted one contains the RX as well as a stimulation and a DSP unit. The external DSP unit is responsible for digitizing and compressing the sound signal from the microphone into coded signals, which are then forwarded from the TX to the RX over the transdermal optical link. In the implanted component, the DSP and stimulation units transform the received signal into a series of electrical pulses that will stimulate the auditory nerve (**Figure 2**). Based on this system model, the performance of the OWCI was evaluated with regard to the SNR, channel capacity, outage probability, and spectral efficiency. The results not only validated the feasibility of the proposed architecture and provided meaningful insights that can be used as design guidelines, but also revealed the superior effectiveness and reliability of the OWCI compared to the conventional CI.

In the aforementioned architecture, the transmitted signal, x, is conveyed over the wireless channel, h, with additive noise n. Thus, the received signal can be written as [68–70].

$$y_1 = Rhx + n \tag{1}$$

with η denoting the quantum efficiency of the photodiode, R the RX's responsivity, v the frequency of the photons, q the electron charge, and p the Planck's constant. It is highlighted that the channel coefficient can be expressed as $h = h_l \; h_p$, where h_l represents the deterministic channel coefficient caused by propagation loss, while h_p denotes the collected power fraction due to the geometric spread from the origin of the detector and is caused from the TX-RX misalignment (**Figure 3**).

The CI channel's deterministic term can be expressed as in ([71], Eq. (10.1))

$$h_l = \exp\left(-(\mu_\alpha(\lambda) + \mu_s(\lambda))\delta\right) \tag{2}$$

where λ is the transmission wavelength, δ is the skin thickness, $\mu_\alpha(\lambda)$ is the skin attenuation coefficient, and $\mu_s(\lambda)$ is the skin scattering coefficient, which can be acquired from a plethora of experimental results [72–76]. In this analysis, the term skin refers to the biological structure that consists from the stratum corneum, the

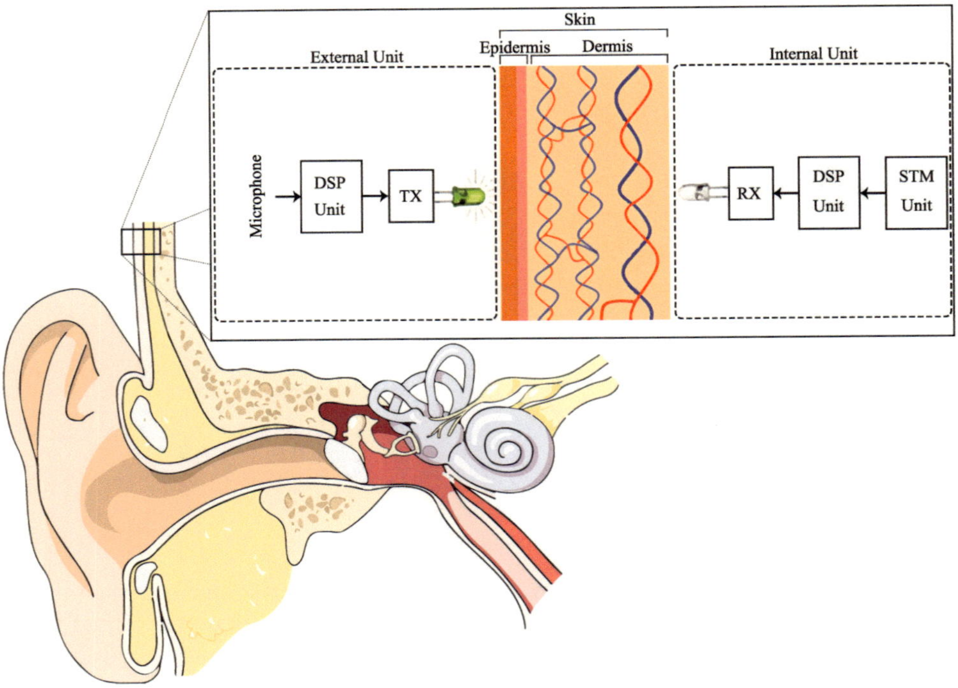

Figure 2.
Diagrammatic illustration of the architecture of the OWCI. The OWCI captures the sound information via the microphone located outside of the human body. Afterward, it utilizes optical wireless communications to transfer it toward the receiver fixed on the cranial bone. Finally, the implanted unit stimulates the acoustic nerve by delivering the appropriate signals via the stimulation electrode.

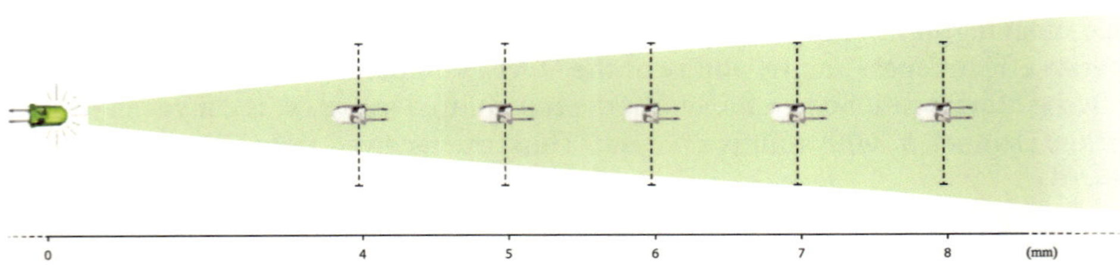

Figure 3.
The effect of misalignment with regard to skin thickness. As the RX (photodiode) moves away from the TX under the same severity of misalignment, its distance from the perfect alignment conditions becomes enclosed in the TX's beam width. This phenomenon creates an equilibrium between the optimal TX-RX distance and the TX beam width under fixed misalignment conditions.

epidermis, and the dermis [71], while both the RX and the TX touch with the inner (adipose) and outer (epidermal) side of the skin [24], and thus, the TX-RX distance is regarded equivalent to skin thickness.

The misalignment between the TX and the RX can be modeled as the stochastic channel coefficient, which expresses the collected power due to geometric spread with radial displacement r from the origin of the detector and can be written as

$$h_p \approx A \exp\left(-\frac{2r^2}{w_e^2}\right), \tag{3}$$

which is based on the assumption that at distance d from the TX, the circular aperture of the transmitted beam has a radius of R and the spatial intensity on the plane of the RX is w_d. In addition, w_e represents the equivalent beam waist radius and A expresses the collected power under perfect alignment. This approximation has been utilized in various previous works for modeling stochastic pointing errors [77, 78].

Based on this model, if we assume independently and identically Gaussian distributed horizontal and vertical displacement, it has been proven that r follows a Rayleigh distribution [79]. As a result, the probability density function (PDF) of the stochastic term of the channel coefficient can be written as

$$f_{h_p}(x) = \frac{\gamma}{A^{\gamma}} x^{\gamma-1}, \qquad 0 \leq x \leq A, \tag{4}$$

where

$$A = (\mathrm{erf}(\beta))^2, \quad \beta = \frac{\sqrt{\pi}R}{\sqrt{2}w_d}, \quad \gamma = \frac{w_e^2}{4\sigma^2}, \quad w_e^2 = w_d^2 \frac{\sqrt{\pi}\mathrm{erf}(\beta)}{2\beta \exp\left(-\beta^2\right)}, \tag{5}$$

while σ^2 denotes the variance of the misalignment.

4.2 All-optical cochlear implant

The CI implementations presented so far counterbalance either the RF scarcity that plagues the communications part of the system or the nerve stimulation limitations. To this end, the AOCI has been proposed as an architecture that converts the audio captured from the microphone into a light signal inside the external component for propagation to the cochlea [17] (**Figure 4**). This way, the AOCI counterbalances the aforementioned challenges and, at the same time, eliminates the need for an energy-consuming DSP unit in the implanted component. The AOCI not only builds upon the fruitful characteristics of the OWCI but also proposes breakthrough alterations such as the fact that it consists of only passive components, and thus, the implanted component has no power demands, which eliminates the requirement of complex power transfer policies and boosts energy efficiency. Furthermore, the AOCI utilizes optical neural stimulation, which is characterized by higher fidelity than electrical neural stimulation due to the lower spread of optical signals in human tissues. The technical advancements include the introduction of the AOCI architecture, its main building blocks, and the end-to-end system model. The AOCI takes into account channel, building block, and biological particularities [17]. Moreover, a novel tractable expression is derived for the instantaneous coupling efficiency in scenarios with misalignment fading. The feasibility of the proposed architecture is proven through the theoretical framework, which also evaluates its performance with regard to the power efficiency, the photon flux, and a plethora of design parameters that greatly influence the success or failure of the system.

Much like OWCI, the architecture of AOCI consists of the implanted and the external component, with the former located on the skull and the latter on the external surface of the skin. The external component captures the acoustic signal with a microphone, performs the necessary DSP, and converts it into the appropriate optical signal capable of generating the desired action potentials on the targeted spiral ganglion neurons. This signal is transmitted from the TX, which is a laser source, to the implanted component, where the guiding lens, the microelectromechanical device,

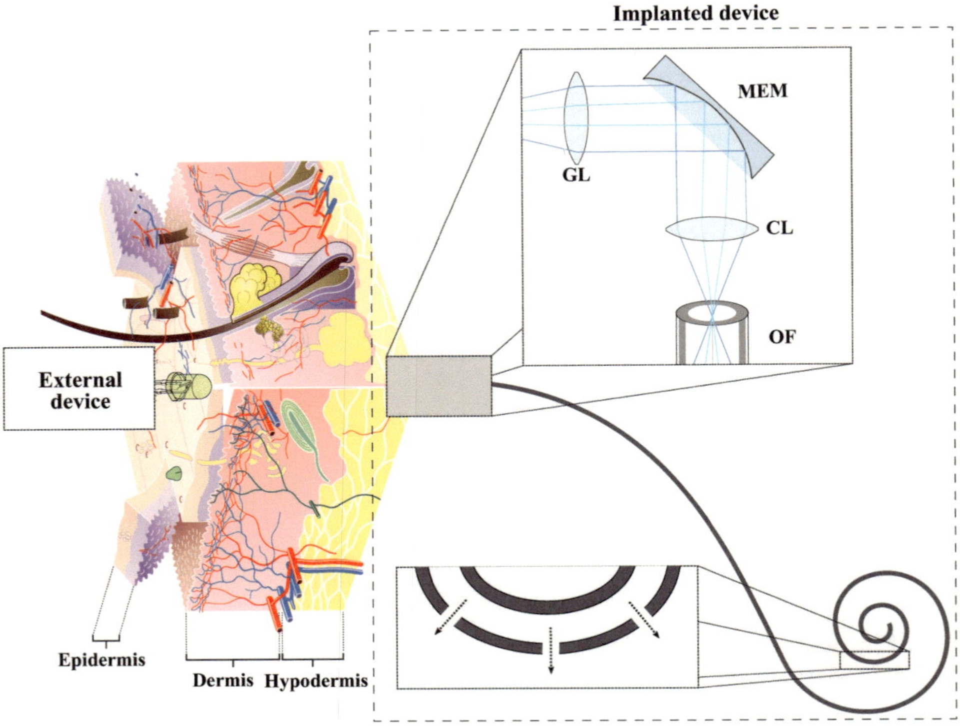

Figure 4.
Illustration of the architecture of the AOCI. The all-optical nature of the AOCI resides in the combined utilization of optical wireless communications and optogenetics for stimulating the auditory nerve. Initially, the auditory neurons are sensitized to optical radiation with optogenetic techniques. Next, the sound captured from the external microphone is converted into an optical signal capable of stimulating the light-sensitive nerves, which is then forwarded to the cochlea.

the coupling lens, and the optical fiber ensure its delivery to the appropriate place in the cochlea. Specifically, the guiding lens guides the light toward the microelectromechanical device to maximize the power of the received optical signal. Afterward, the microelectromechanical acts as a mirror that mitigates the misalignment to a degree by steering the light beam to the center of the coupling lens in order to be coupled into the optical fiber. Finally, the latter delivers the light into specific points along the cochlea based on their spectral content.

4.2.1 Microelectromechanical device

Microelectromechanical devices have been the subject of much hype during the past decade due to their adaptability as well as low cost, low weight, and small size [80–82]. In the case of the AOCI, the microelectromechanical device is required in order to account for the individuality of each patient. In particular, the AOCI is required to adapt to the particularities of the patient, such as different skin thickness and color or slightly varied orientation of biological tissues, in order to ensure uninterrupted hearing restoration. Moreover, imperfections during the implantation process can cause slight variations to the final placement of the implant. To this end, the microelectromechanical device provides an externally operated light control system by enabling the steering of the optical beam toward the coupling lens. Finally, the microelectromechanical device adjusts its optical properties and, thus, steers the beam after receiving the appropriate electrical charge that can be applied during implantation, while in normal operation, the need for adjustment is eliminated, and therefore, the microelectromechanical device operates passively [83, 84].

The signal received by the guiding lens presented in (1) is forwarded to the microelectromechanical device, which introduces a collimation gain [85].

$$G_c = \frac{1}{\sqrt{(1 - d_{in}/f)^2 + z_0^2/f^2}}. \tag{6}$$

Therefore, the updated received signal at the output of the microelectromechanical device can be expressed as

$$y_2 = G_c h_l h_p x + n. \tag{7}$$

4.2.2 Coupling lens

The coupling lens receives the optical beam from the microelectromechanical device and focuses it in the center of the optical fiber. The fact that incident light on the end of the optical fiber that arrives at a greater angle than the acceptable angle of the optical fiber is not coupled highlights the detrimental impact it plays on the maximum achievable coupling efficiency of the system. Moreover, the coupling efficiency is also affected by the dimensions of the coupling lens and the diameter of the optical fiber with its maximum value being in the order of 80% [86].

The coupling lens captures the optical signal that is reflected by the microelectromechanical device and couples it into the optical fiber. The signal that successfully enters the optical fiber can be written as

$$y_3 = \eta G_c h_l h_p x + n \tag{8}$$

with the coupling efficiency given by

$$\eta = \left(\frac{3.83\sqrt{2}D\omega_0}{1.22\lambda F} \exp\left(-\frac{r^2}{\omega_0^2}\right)\Psi_2\left(1; 2, 1; -\frac{3.83^2 D^2 \omega_0^2}{1.22^2 \lambda^2 F^2}, \frac{r^2}{\omega_0^2}\right)\right)^2. \tag{9}$$

In Eq. (9), ω_0, F, D, and ρ denote the optical fiber mode field radius, the focal length, the focusing lens diameter, and the radial distance on the focal plane, respectively, while it becomes obvious that the achievable coupling efficiency is dependent on the optical fiber's mode field radius, the coupling lens's focal length and diameter, as well as the intensity of misalignment and the transmission wavelength.

4.2.3 Optical fiber

The optical fiber of the AOCI takes the place of the electrode array of the conventional CI. The incident optical signal must be delivered to specific locations alongside the cochlea in order to generate action potentials at the targeted spiral ganglion neurons that are responsible for the appropriate sound frequency. To achieve the required performance, the optical fiber proposed in the AOCI architecture propagates the optical signal through its single-mode core with a Gaussian beam profile in the output [87, 88]. Furthermore, despite the fact that state-of-the-art conventional CIs can be equipped with a maximum of 20 electrodes, due to the limited spatial resolution of electrical neural stimulation, the sound perceived by the patient has the fidelity of eight functional electrodes [40]. In addition, to achieve speech and music perception under suboptimal noise constraints, CI must house approximately 32 electrodes, which is also the goal of the AOCI [89, 90]. Therefore, tilted fiber Bragg gratings (FBGs) were introduced in the AOCI architecture that enable light delivery in various locations alongside the optical fiber [91, 92]. These FBGs are located in the core of the optical fiber, along the propagation direction, with a periodic variation of the refractive index. These components have low insertion loss, low complexity structures, and high wavelength selectivity. Specifically, tilted FBGs allow a limited number of wavelengths to penetrate them by filtering the incident optical signal based on its spectral content and, at the time, redirecting it based to their angle [93, 94].

When the optical signal travels through the optical fiber, it attenuates due to the curvature of the optical fiber and the existence of FBGs, and therefore, the emitted signal can be expressed as

$$y_4 = k\eta G_c h_l h_p x + n, \tag{10}$$

where k denotes the propagation efficiency, which is limited to $0.14\,\mathrm{dB}/90^{\circ}$ by the strong optical confinement of microfiber, even for increased bending radius or index values [95]. In addition, k incorporates the signal attenuation due to the existence of FBGs, which has been proven to be in the order of 10% [96].

5. The road ahead

From the presented analysis, it is evident that, despite their extensive applications, electrical neural stimulation techniques suffer from insufficient coding of spectral information, low power efficiency, low stimulation precision, accuracy, and frequency, as well as questionable safety. To this end, promising optical neural stimulation methods that surpass these limitations have been proposed. In an effort to establish these methods, the scientific community has pushed toward proving their feasibility as well as theoretically modeling and augmenting them. The state of the art of optical neural stimulation techniques offers great promise toward realizing next-generation biomedical systems.

One of the main offerings of optical neural stimulation is the outstanding stimulation precision it offers compared to electrical neural stimulation. In more detail, the increased precision can be translated into higher customization of the produced neural activity in two respects. First, the increased stimulation frequency that comes with optical neural stimulation leads to higher accuracy of excitation due to the fact that action potentials are delivered faster to the target spiral ganglion neurons and, therefore, to the brain, thus limiting the time between sound acquisition and perception. Second, optical neural stimulation depends on the optical particularities of light sensitive opsins with each one being expressed in a specific type of cell. Therefore, this offers another layer of light selectivity that can be leveraged by optical neural stimulation techniques [97]. The combination of these two aspects equips optical neural stimulation with the necessary tools to achieve unprecedented performance not only in the field of hearing restoration but also in other biomedical application such as retinal implants that would utilize this advantage to provide higher perceived image fidelity.

Another aspect that boosts the performance of optical neural stimulation is the exceptional spectral coding of the information carried by the optical signal. On the contrary to electrical neural stimulation techniques that are characterized by wide current spread from the electrode contacts, optical radiation attenuates with a greater rate when it propagates inside human tissue, and therefore, the applied optical stimulations are more spatially confined than electrical ones. The importance of this phenomenon is highlighted even more by the fact that human sound perception requires at least 32 stimulation channels in order to recognize music or sound in noisy environments [89, 90]. As a result, the superior spectral coding of optical neural stimulation enables support for stimulation units that can house significantly more channels.

Contrary to previous detrimental improvements offered by optical neural stimulation methods, their performance in terms of power efficiency is comparable to the one of electrical neural stimulation. In more detail, optimization is required for optical neural stimulation stimulation policies in order to achieve similar power consumption as electrical neural stimulation [58]. Therefore, the optimization of optical neural stimulation techniques in terms of their power demands is one of the key requirements for their successful application in future biomedical applications. Similarly, the safety and ethical concerns of optical neural stimulation pose another controversial aspect. On the one hand, the optical power that is required for the reliable activation of light-sensitive spiral ganglion neurons is below the limits defined in various standardization protocols [98]; on the other hand, the modification of the targeted spiral ganglion neurons in order to acquire light sensitivity poses ethical concerns.

From a purely biological perspective, action potentials generated from electrical stimulation signals resemble the morphology and waveform of the membrane potential. As a result, these electrical signals are superimposed on each other and become almost indistinguishable, which hinders hearing restoration [58]. However, owing to its core functionality, optical neural stimulation triggers action potentials that differ significantly from membrane potential based on the stimulation protocol and the type of the excited cell. Specifically, not only the waveform of the generated action potential is affected by the amplitude and the duration of the stimulation, but also the instant release of ions when opsins are illuminated, which causes the membrane to react immediately. In addition, each opsin-cell-type combination is characterized by a distinct morphology of transmembrane potential and in conjunction with the wide variety of opsins available; they ensure the generation of a distinct action potential.

Finally, from an engineering point of view, the plethora of opsins that have been developed can highly impact the performance of optical neural stimulation biomedical applications. All future research in this field should take into careful consideration the selection of the applied opsin, as suboptimal ones may result in low stimulation precision and reliability, which, in turn, can determine whether the application is successful or not. The most important design choices include the compatibility with the target cell type, the amplitude and morphology of the resulting action potential, and the nature and the direction of the released ions.

6. Conclusions

In this chapter, we have provided a vision for hearing restoration from an engineering point of view that could serve as a guide in the research and development of the next-generation CIs. We suggest that the future of digital hearing restoration lies in the optical spectrum, both in terms of communication and stimulation techniques.

We envisioned and explained potential architectures that enable the utilization of optical technologies in CIs. Finally, we introduced key features and performance indicators that could decide their success or failure.

Conflict of interest

The authors declare no conflict of interest.

Nomenclature

AOCI	all-optical cochlear implant
BER	bit error rate
ChR2	channelrhodopsin 2
CI	cochlear implant
DSP	digital signal processing
FBG	fiber Bragg grating
LED	light-emitting diode
MPE	maximum permissible exposure
OWCI	optical wireless cochlear implant
RF	radio frequency
SNR	signal-to-noise ratio

Author details

Stylianos E. Trevlakis[1], Alexandros-Apostolos A. Boulogeorgos[2]* and George K. Karagiannidis[1]

1 Department of Electrical and Computer Engineering, Aristotle University of Thessaloniki, Thessaloniki, Greece

2 Department of Digital Systems, University of Piraeus, Piraeus, Greece

*Address all correspondence to: al.boulogeorgos@ieee.org

References

[1] Moser T, Grabner CP, Schmitz F. Sensory processing at ribbon synapses in the retina and the cochlea. Physiological Reviews. 2020;**100**(1):103-144

[2] Deafness and Hearing Loss. Available from: https://www.who.int/news-room/fact-sheets/detail/deafness-and-hearing-loss

[3] Samarajeewa A, Jacques BE, Dabdoub A. Therapeutic potential of Wnt and Notch signaling and epigenetic regulation in mammalian sensory hair cell regeneration. Molecular Therapy. 2019;**27**(5):904-911

[4] Roccio M, Senn P, Heller S. Novel insights into inner ear development and regeneration for targeted hearing loss therapies. Hearing Restoration. 2020; **397**:107859

[5] Miller CA, Abbas PJ, Robinson BK, Nourski KV, Zhang F, Jeng FC. Electrical excitation of the acoustically sensitive auditory nerve: Single-fiber responses to electric pulse trains. Journal of the Association for Research in Otolaryngology. 2006;7(3):195-210

[6] Caldwell MT, Jiam NT, Limb CJ. Assessment and improvement of sound quality in cochlear implant users. Laryngoscope Investigative Otolaryngology. 2017;**2**(3):119-124

[7] Djourno A, Eyries C. Auditory prosthesis by means of a distant electrical stimulation of the sensory nerve with the use of an indwelt coiling. La Presse Médicale. 1957;**65**:1417

[8] House WF, Urban J. Long term results of electrode implantation and electronic stimulation of the cochlea in man. The Annals of Otology, Rhinology, and Laryngology. 1973;**82**(4):504-517

[9] Burian K. Letter: Significance of cochlear nerve electric stimulation in totally deaf patients. Laryngologie, Rhinologie, Otologie. 1975;**54**:530-531

[10] Trevlakis SE, Boulogeorgos AAA, Karagiannidis GK. On the impact of misalignment fading in transdermal optical wireless communications. In: 2018 7th International Conference on Modern Circuits and Systems Technologies (MOCAST). Thessaloniki, Greece: IEEE; 2018

[11] Trevlakis SE, Boulogeorgos AAA, Sofotasios PC, Muhaidat S, Karagiannidis GK. Optical wireless cochlear implants. Biomedical Optics Express. 2019;**10**(2):707

[12] Izzo AD, Walsh JT, Jansen ED, Bendett M, Webb J, Ralph H, et al. Optical parameter variability in laser nerve stimulation: A study of pulse duration, repetition rate, and wavelength. IEEE Transactions on Biomedical Engineering. 2007;**54**(6): 1108-1114

[13] Moser T. Optogenetic stimulation of the auditory pathway for research and future prosthetics. Current Opinion in Neurobiology. 2015;**34**:29-36

[14] Jeschke M, Moser T. Considering optogenetic stimulation for cochlear implants. Hearing Research. 2015;**322**: 224-234

[15] Trevlakis SE, Boulogeorgos AAA, Chatzidiamantis ND, Karagiannidis GK, Lei X. Electrical vs optical cell stimulation: A communication perspective. IEEE Access. 2020;**8**: 192259-192269

[16] Baumhoff P, Kallweit N, Kral A. Intracochlear near infrared stimulation:

Feasibility of optoacoustic stimulation in vivo. Hearing Research. 2019;**371**: 40-52

[17] Trevlakis SE, Boulogeorgos AAA, Chatzidiamantis ND, Karagiannidis GK. All-optical Cochlear implants. IEEE Transactions on Molecular, Biological and Multi-Scale Communications. 2020; **6**(1):13-24

[18] Zeng FG, Rebscher S, Harrison W, Sun X, Feng H. Cochlear implants: System design, integration, and evaluation. IEEE Reviews in Biomedical Engineering. 2008;**1**:115-142

[19] Agarwal K, Jegadeesan R, Guo YX, Thakor NV. Wireless power transfer strategies for implantable bioelectronics. IEEE Reviews in Biomedical Engineering. 2017;**10**:136-161

[20] Kim HJ, Hirayama H, Kim S, Han KJ, Zhang R, Choi JW. Review of near-field wireless power and communication for biomedical applications. IEEE Access. 2017;**5**:21264-21285

[21] Thompson AC, Wade SA, Pawsey NC, Stoddart PR. Infrared neural stimulation: Influence of stimulation site spacing and repetition rates on heating. IEEE Transactions on Biomedical Engineering. 2013;**60**(12):3534-3541

[22] Ko WH. Early history and challenges of implantable electronics. Journal on Emerging Technologies in Computing Systems. 2012;**8**(2):1-9

[23] Islam MN, Yuce MR. Review of medical implant communication system (MICS) band and network. ICT Express. 2016;**2**(4):188-194

[24] Liu T, Bihr U, Anis SM, Ortmanns M. Optical transcutaneous link for low power, high data rate telemetry. In: Annual International Conference of the IEEE Engineering in Medicine and Biology Society (EMBC). San Diego, CA, USA: IEEE; 2012. pp. 3535-3538

[25] Pinski SL, Trohman RG. Interference in implanted cardiac devices, Part I. Pacing and Clinical Electrophysiology. 2002;**25**(9):1367-1381

[26] Dieter A, Keppeler D, Moser T. Towards the optical cochlear implant: Optogenetic approaches for hearing restoration. Molecular Medicine. 2020;**12** (4):e11618

[27] Wrobel C, Dieter A, Huet A, Keppeler D, Duque-Afonso CJ, Vogl C, et al. Optogenetic stimulation of cochlear neurons activates the auditory pathway and restores auditory-driven behavior in deaf adult gerbils. Science Translational Medicine. 2018;**10**(449): eaao0540

[28] Keppeler D, Merino RM, de la Morena DL, Bali B, Huet AT, Gehrt A, et al. Ultrafast optogenetic stimulation of the auditory pathway by targeting-optimized Chronos. The EMBO Journal. 2018;**37**(24):e99649

[29] Mager T, de la Morena DL, Senn V, Schlotte J, Feldbauer K, Wrobel C, et al. High frequency neural spiking and auditory signaling by ultrafast red-shifted optogenetics. Nature Communications. 2018;**9**(1):1750

[30] Ghassemlooy Z, Alves LN, Zvanovec S, Khalighi MA. Visible Light Communications: Theory and Applications. Boca Raton: CRC Press; 2017

[31] Chowdhury MZ, Hossan MT, Islam A, Jang YM. A comparative survey of optical wireless technologies: Architectures and applications. IEEE Access. 2018;**6**:9819-9840

[32] Abita JL, Schneider W. Transdermal optical communications. Johns Hopkins APL Technical Digest. 2004;**25**(3):261

[33] Ackermann DM Jr, Smith B, Wang XF, Kilgore KL, Peckham PH. Designing the optical interface of a transcutaneous optical telemetry link. IEEE Transactions on Biomedical Engineering. 2008;**55**(4):1365-1373

[34] Gil Y, Rotter N, Arnon S. Feasibility of retroreflective transdermal optical wireless communication. Applied Optics. 2002;**51**(18):4232-4239

[35] Liu T, Anders J, Ortmanns M. Bidirectional optical transcutaneous telemetric link for brain machine interface. Electronics Letters. 2015; **51**(24):1969-1971

[36] Duncan K, Etienne-Cummings R. Selecting a safe power level for an indoor implanted UWB wireless biotelemetry link. In: IEEE Biomedical Circuits and Systems Conference (BioCAS). Rotterdam, Netherlands: IEEE; 2013. pp. 230-233

[37] Ackermann DM, Smith B, Kilgore KL, Peckham PH. Design of a high speed transcutaneous optical telemetry link. In: Engineering in Medicine and Biology Society, 2006. EMBS'06. 28th Annual International Conference of the IEEE. New York, NY, USA: IEEE; 2006. pp. 2932-2935

[38] Liu T, Anders J, Ortmanns M. System level model for transcutaneous optical telemetric link. In: IEEE International Symposium on Circuits and Systems (ISCAS). Beijing, China: IEEE; 2013. pp. 865-868

[39] Luan S, Williams I, Nikolic K, Constandinou TG. Neuromodulation: Present and emerging methods. Frontiers in Neuroengineering. 2014;7:27

[40] Srinivasan AG, Landsberger DM, Shannon RV. Current focusing sharpens local peaks of excitation in cochlear implant stimulation. Hearing Research. 2010;**270**(1–2):89-100

[41] Hardesty DE, Sackeim HA. Deep brain stimulation in movement and psychiatric disorders. Biological Psychiatry. 2007;**61**(7):831-835

[42] Rosellini WM, Yoo PB, Engineer N, Armstrong S, Weiner RL, Burress C, et al. A voltage-controlled capacitive discharge method for electrical activation of peripheral nerves. Neuromodulation: Technology at the Neural Interface. 2011;**14**(6):493-500

[43] Wong LSY, Hossain S, Ta A, Edvinsson J, Rivas DH, Naas H. A very low-power CMOS mixed-signal IC for implantable pacemaker applications. IEEE Journal of Solid-State Circuits. 2004;**39**(12):2446-2456

[44] Foutz TJ Jr, DMA, Kilgore KL, McIntyre CC. Energy efficient neural stimulation: Coupling circuit design and membrane biophysics. PLoS One. 2012; 7(12):e51901

[45] Sahin M, Tie Y. Non-rectangular waveforms for neural stimulation with practical electrodes. Journal of Neural Engineering. 2007;**4**(3):227-233

[46] Albensi BC, Oliver DR, Toupin J, Odero G. Electrical stimulation protocols for hippocampal synaptic plasticity and neuronal hyper-excitability: Are they effective or relevant? Experimental Neurology. 2007;**204**(1):1-13

[47] Yip M, Bowers P, Noel V, Chandrakasan A, Stankovic KM. Energy-efficient waveform for electrical stimulation of the cochlear nerve. Scientific Reports. 2017;**7**(1):13582

[48] Aravanis AM, Wang LP, Zhang F, Meltzer LA, Mogri MZ, Schneider MB, et al. An optical neural interface: in vivocontrol of rodent motor cortex with integrated fiberoptic and optogenetic technology. Journal of Neural Engineering. 2007;**4**(3):S143-S156

[49] Adamantidis AR, Zhang F, Aravanis AM, Deisseroth K, de Lecea L. Neural substrates of awakening probed with optogenetic control of hypocretin neurons. Nature. 2007;**450**(7168):420-424

[50] Petreanu L, Mao T, Sternson SM, Svoboda K. The subcellular organization of neocortical excitatory connections. Nature. 2009;**457**(7233):1142-1145

[51] Lin JY, Sann SB, Zhou K, Nabavi S, Proulx CD, Malinow R, et al. Optogenetic inhibition of synaptic release with chromophore-assisted light inactivation (CALI). Neuron. 2013;**79**(2):241-253

[52] Renault R, Sukenik N, Descroix S, Malaquin L, Viovy JL, Peyrin JM, et al. Combining microfluidics, optogenetics and calcium imaging to study neuronal communication in vitro. PLoS One. 2015; **10**(4):e0120680

[53] Schmid F, Wachsmuth L, Schwalm M, Prouvot PH, Jubal ER, Fois C, et al. Assessing sensory versus optogenetic network activation by combining (o)fMRI with optical Ca2+ recordings. Journal of Cerebral Blood Flow & Metabolism. 2016; **36**(11):1885-1900

[54] Nagel G, Szellas T, Huhn W, Kateriya S, Adeishvili N, Berthold P, et al. Channelrhodopsin-2, a directly light-gated cation-selective membrane channel. Proceedings of the National Academy of Sciences. 2003;**100**(24): 13940-13945

[55] Entcheva E. Cardiac optogenetics. American Journal of Physiology-Heart and Circulatory Physiology. 2013; **304**(9):H1179-H1191

[56] Jiang C, Li HT, Zhou YM, Wang X, Wang L, Liu ZQ. Cardiac optogenetics: A novel approach to cardiovascular disease therapy. EP Europace. 2017;**20**: 1741-1749

[57] O'Shea C, Holmes AP, Winter J, Correia J, Ou X, Dong R, et al. Cardiac optogenetics and optical mapping—Overcoming spectral congestion in all-optical cardiac electrophysiology. Frontiers in Physiology. 2019;**10**:182

[58] Williams JC, Entcheva E. Optogenetic versus electrical stimulation of human cardiomyocytes: Modeling insights. Biophysical Journal. 2015; **108**(8):1934-1945

[59] Boyden E. A history of optogenetics: The development of tools for controlling brain circuits with light. F1000 Biology Reports. 2011;**3**:11

[60] Yizhar O, Fenno LE, Davidson TJ, Mogri M, Deisseroth K. Optogenetics in neural systems. Neuron. 2011;**71**(1):9-34

[61] Gunaydin LA, Yizhar O, Berndt A, Sohal VS, Deisseroth K, Hegemann P. Ultrafast optogenetic control. Nature Neuroscience. 2010;**13**(3):387-392

[62] Berndt A, Schoenenberger P, Mattis J, Tye KM, Deisseroth K, Hegemann P, et al. High-efficiency channelrhodopsins for fast neuronal stimulation at low light levels. Proceedings of the National Academy of Sciences. 2011;**108**(18):7595-7600

[63] Goßler C, Bierbrauer C, Moser R, Kunzer M, Holc K, Pletschen W, et al. GaN-based micro-LED arrays on flexible substrates for optical cochlear implants. Journal of Physics D: Applied Physics. 2014;**47**(20):205401. Available from:

http://stacks.iop.org/0022-3727/47/i=20/a=205401

[64] Kallweit N, Baumhoff P, Krueger A, Tinne N, Kral A, Ripken T, et al. Optoacoustic effect is responsible for laser-induced cochlear responses. Scientific Reports. 2016;**6**(28141):1-10

[65] Schultz M, Baumhoff P, Kallweit N, Sato M, Krüger A, Ripken T, et al. Optical stimulation of the hearing and deaf cochlea under thermal and stress confinement condition. In: Optical Techniques in Neurosurgery, Neurophotonics, and Optogenetics. International Society for Optics and Photonics. San Francisco, California, United States: SPIE; 2014. p. 892816

[66] Richter CP, Tan X. Photons and neurons. Hearing Research. 2014;**311** (Supplement C):72-88. Annual Reviews

[67] Duke AR, Cayce JM, Malphrus JD, Konrad P, Mahadevan-Jansen A, Jansen ED. Combined optical and electrical stimulation of neural tissue in vivo. Journal of Biomedical Optics. 2009;**14**(6):060501-060501

[68] Li J, Uysal M. Optical wireless communications: System model, capacity and coding. In: IEEE 58th Vehicular Technology Conference. VTC 2003-Fall (IEEE Cat. No.03CH37484). Vol. 1. Orlando, FL, USA: IEEE; 2003. pp. 168-172

[69] Zedini E, Alouini MS. Multihop relaying over IM/DD FSO systems with pointing errors. Journal of Lightwave Technology. 2015;**33**(23):5007-5015

[70] Popoola WO, Ghassemlooy Z. BPSK subcarrier intensity modulated free-space optical communications in atmospheric turbulence. Journal of Lightwave Technology. 2009;**27**(8): 967-973

[71] Faria M, Alves LN, de Brito André PS. 10. In: Transdermal Optical Communications. Vol. 1. Boca Raton: CRC Press; 2017. pp. 309-336.

[72] Bashkatov AN, Genina EA, Tuchin VV. Optical properties of skin, subcutaneous, and muscle tissues: A review. Journal of Innovative Optical Health Sciences. 2011;**4**(01):9-38

[73] Simpson CR, Kohl M, Essenpreis M, Cope M. Near-infrared optical properties of ex-vivo human skin and subcutaneous tissues measured using the Monte Carlo inversion technique. Physics in Medicine and Biology. 1998;**43**(9):2465

[74] Du Y, Hu X, Cariveau M, Ma X, Kalmus G, Lu J. Optical properties of porcine skin dermis between 900 nm and 1500 nm. Physics in Medicine and Biology. 2001;**46**(1):167

[75] Troy TL, Thennadil SN. Optical properties of human skin in the near infrared wavelength range of 1000 to 2200 nm. Journal of Biomedical Optics. 2001;**6**(2):167-176

[76] Bashkatov A, Genina E, Kochubey V, Tuchin V. Optical properties of human skin, subcutaneous and mucous tissues in the wavelength range from 400 to 2000 nm. Journal of Physics D: Applied Physics. 2005;**38**(15):2543

[77] Farid AA, Hranilovic S. Outage capacity optimization for free-space optical links with pointing errors. Journal of Lightwave Technology. 2007;**25**(7): 1702-1710

[78] Sandalidis HG, Tsiftsis TA, Karagiannidis GK, Uysal M. BER performance of FSO links over strong atmospheric turbulence channels with pointing errors. IEEE Communications Letters. 2008;**12**(1): 44-46

[79] Arnon S. Effects of atmospheric turbulence and building sway on optical wireless-communication systems. Optics Letters. 2003;**28**(2):129-131

[80] Zou Y, Zhang W, Tian F, Chau FS, Zhou G. Development of miniature tunable multi-element Alvarez lenses. IEEE Journal of Selected Topics in Quantum Electronics. 2015;**21**(4): 100-107

[81] Hwang K, Seo YH, Jeong KH. Microscanners for optical endomicroscopic applications. Micro and Nano Systems Letters. 2017;**5**(1): 2213-9621

[82] Zhou G, Lee C, editors. Optical MEMS, Nanophotonics, and their Applications. Boca Raton: CRC Press; 2017

[83] Khoshnoud F, de Silva CW. Recent advances in MEMS sensor technology—Biomedical applications. IEEE Instrumentation & Measurement Magazine. 2012;**15**(1):8-14

[84] Sezen AS, Sivaramakrishnan S, Hur S, Rajamani R, Robbins W, Nelson BJ. Passive wireless MEMS microphones for biomedical applications. Journal of Biomechanical Engineering. 2005;**127**(6):1030-1034

[85] Sabry Y, Khalil D, Saadany B, Bourouina T. In-plane optical beam collimation using a three-dimensional curved MEMS mirror. Micromachines. 2017;**8**(5):134

[86] Nguyen H, Arnob MMP, Becker AT, Wolfe JC, Hogan MK, Horner PJ, et al. Fabrication of multipoint side-firing optical fiber by laser micro-ablation. Optics Letters. 2017;**42**(9):1808-1811

[87] Wells JD, Xing A, Bendett MP, Keller MD, Norton BJ, Owen JM, et al. Laser-based nerve stimulators for, EG, hearing restoration in cochlear prostheses and method. Google Patents; 2014. US Patent 8.792.978

[88] Marcuse D. Gaussian approximation of the fundamental modes of graded-index fibers. Journal of the Optical Society of America. 1978;**68**(1):103

[89] Friesen LM, Shannon RV, Baskent D, Wang X. Speech recognition in noise as a function of the number of spectral channels: Comparison of acoustic hearing and cochlear implants. The Journal of the Acoustical Society of America. 2001;**110**(2):1150-1163

[90] Kong YY, Cruz R, Jones JA, Zeng FG. Music perception with temporal cues in acoustic and electric hearing. Ear and Hearing. 2004;**25**(2): 173-185

[91] Zhou K, Zhang L, Chen X, Bennion I. Optic sensors of high refractive-index responsivity and low thermal cross sensitivity that use fiber Bragg gratings of $> 80^{\circ}$ tilted structures. Optics Letters. 2006;**31**(9):1193-1195

[92] Cotillard R, Laffont G, Ferdinand P. Regeneration of tilted fiber Bragg gratings. In: 23rd International Conference on Optical Fibre Sensors. Santander, Spain: SPIE; 2014. p. 91572S

[93] Bharathan G, Hudson DD, Woodward RI, Jackson SD, Fuerbach A. In-fiber polarizer based on a 45-degree tilted fluoride fiber Bragg grating for mid-infrared fiber laser technology. OSA Continuum. 2018;**1**(1):56-63

[94] Mou C, Zhou K, Zhang L, Bennion I. Characterization of 45°-tilted fiber grating and its polarization function in fiber ring laser. Journal of the Optical Society of America B: Optical Physics. 2009;**26**(10):1905

[95] Yu H, Wang S, Fu J, Qiu M, Li Y, Gu F, et al. Modeling bending losses of optical nanofibers or nanowires. Applied Optics. 2009;**48**(22):4365-4369

[96] Wang G, Wang C, Yan Z, Zhang L. Highly efficient spectrally encoded imaging using a 45° tilted fiber grating. Optics Letters. 2016;**41**(11):2398

[97] Cardin JA, Carlén M, Meletis K, Knoblich U, Zhang F, Deisseroth K, et al. Driving fast-spiking cells induces gamma rhythm and controls sensory responses. Nature. 2009;**459**(7247): 663-667

[98] International Commission on Non-Ionizing Radiation Protection. ICNIRP guidelines on limits of exposure to laser radiation of wavelengths between 180 nm and 1,000 μm. Health Physics. 2013; **105**(3):271-295